yoga
for
mother
and baby

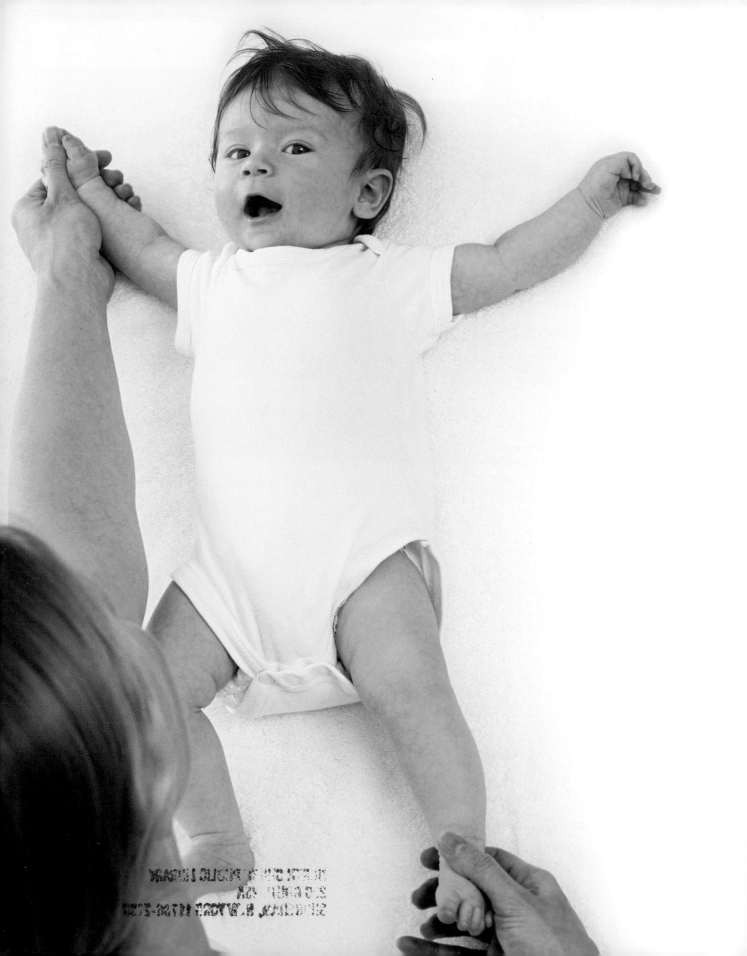

yoga
for
mother
and baby

Julie Llewellyn-Thomas

photography by Ruth Jenkinson

MITCHELL BEAZLEY

For my children – Clara, Rafi, Gabriel, and baby Lucia

First published in Great Britain in 2006 by Mitchell Beazley
An imprint of Octopus Publishing Group Ltd,
2–4 Heron Quays, Docklands, London E14 4JP

The views and advice expressed in this book are those of the author and based on her expertise and experience as a practising yoga teacher and mother, having worked with new mothers and babies aged between 6 weeks and 12 months with the yoga techniques described. While the advice and information in this book is believed to be accurate and true at the time of going to press, no legal responsibility or liability can be accepted by the Publisher for any errors or omissions that may be made. This book is not intended as a substitute for professional medical advice where necessary and appropriate. As with any exercise programme it is advisable for the reader to consult with their medical practitioner and/or health visitor in all matters relating to the health of themselves and their baby and particularly in respect of any symptoms which may requre diagnosis or medical attention prior to embarking on any exercise programme.

ISBN 1 84533 173 7

A CIP record for this book is
available from the British Library

To order this book as a gift or incentive contact Mitchell Beazley on 020 7531 8481

Typeset in Perpetua
Produced by Toppan Printing Co., (HK) Ltd
Printed and bound in China

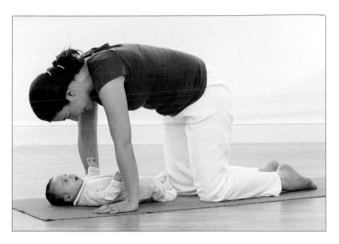

CONTENTS

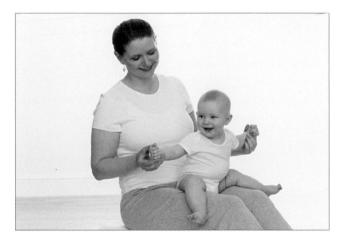

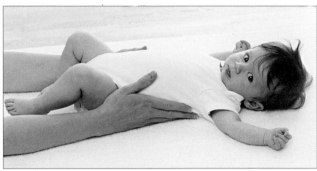

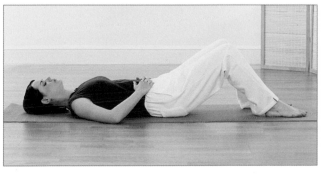

What is yoga?

The practice of yoga can bring many rewards: it will awaken your body, sharpen your mind, and clarify your spirit. You can decide how deeply involved with yoga you want to be. It may form just a small part of your routine or you may wish to incorporate its theories, postures, diet, and philosophy into every aspect of your life. But you will find that simply practising these exercises with your baby will begin to transform the way you feel, move, breathe, and interact with your baby and those around you.

Yoga has been described as the oldest form of personal development known to humankind, dating back some 5000 years. Although originally it was performed only by men – not until the 20th century did Indian yoga schools begin to admit women – today yoga has spread around the world and is practised by people of all abilities and ages, by both the sick and the healthy.

Yoga is derived from the Sanskrit word "yug", meaning "union", and the essence of yoga is a yoking together of mind, body, and spirit. Its combination of postures, breath control, and meditation can promote relaxation and a sense of fulfilment or spirituality, although yoga is not a religion as such.

Practising yoga will benefit you, your baby, and your relationship together. Yoga is non-competitive and is not a sport, so don't worry if you wouldn't describe yourself as athletic – it is important that you learn to work at your own level without straining.

Simple yoga exercises can help a baby's balance, improve coordination and motor skills, and aid the respiratory and digestive systems, and babies who practise yoga are less likely to suffer colic and constipation. Yoga also allows babies to move freely – a welcome release from the restraints of a car seat or carry cot. Practising yoga as a mother will help you to relax and feel emotionally focused and supported, and you and your baby will share physical and spiritual bonds as you practise yoga together.

Baby yoga is an extension of baby massage, which has been practised in many cultures for centuries. Around the world, massage has been used to ease childbirth, aid recovery, stimulate and soothe babies, and alleviate a range of adult ailments. In many societies, massage for both mother and baby is a part of traditional birthing practice and new-born babies are massaged to stimulate their survival mechanisms and help them resist disease.

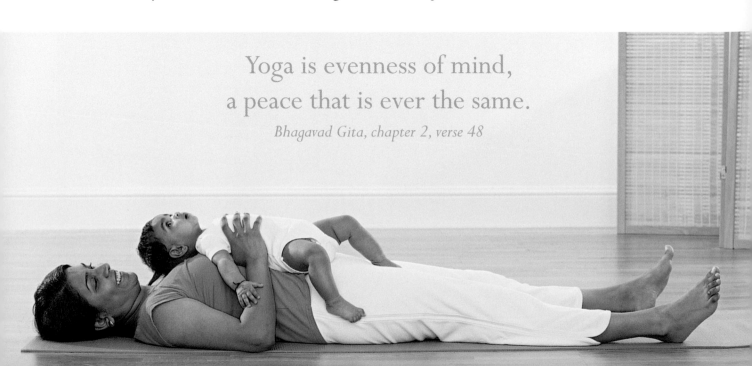

Yoga is evenness of mind,
a peace that is ever the same.

Bhagavad Gita, chapter 2, verse 48

Yoga is an ideal form of exercise to practise during the postnatal period. It is diverse enough to contain a huge range of physical levels, from gentle movements to vigorous exercise. After the birth you will be facing many adjustments to your life and may feel both joy and despair, as well as tiredness and frustration with your appearance. The deep relaxed breathing promoted by yoga can fill your body with "prana" (energy), while the calm, supine posture of "shavasana" will recharge you, leaving you better able to direct your body's resources toward healing yourself and caring for your baby.

Yoga and the breath cannot be separated – in yogic terms, a life is measured not in years but in the number of breaths you take. By learning to breathe correctly, you will learn to calm your mind and emotions – there is evidence of an intrinsic link between the emotions and the breath. You will notice that if you are angry or tense you breathe quickly and in a shallow way. By slowing down and deepening your breathing, you will find that you will begin to calm yourself down and feel more relaxed.

Yoga brings mindfulness: it teaches us to focus on the here and now and to appreciate life's gifts and helps us to face its difficulties with clarity and openness. Yoga can offer a grounding in parenting, teaching us to enjoy the moment yet be always open to reflection. As we learn to care for ourselves, gain an understanding of our own needs and limitations, forgive our mistakes, and be open to improvement, we will be better equipped to parent in an honest way, without feeling spiritually or emotionally parched.

There are various branches of yoga, of which Hatha yoga, based on physical movements and postures called "asanas", is the most popular and widely known. Hatha yoga, which has found a strong following in Western society over the past decades, is also regarded as "traditional" yoga and provides the basis for the practices in this book.

Asanas can be combined in different ways, meeting a number of muscular, meditative, and energetic needs. They also encourage concentration on the connection between breathing, the physical self, thoughts, and feelings. "Hatha" is formed from the Sanskrit words for the sun and moon, indicating a fusion of opposites, but Hatha yoga can equally be understood as "yoga of activity". Hatha yoga is practical, relaxing muscles and improving posture, strength, and flexibility. It is also slow paced and gentle, calming and meditative, using breathing techniques, or "Pranyama", to improve health. But for you and your baby, yoga can most especially bring joy, fulfilment, and a greater sense of togetherness.

THE YOGA SUTRAS

You may want to learn more about the eight limbs of yoga described in Patanjali's *Yoga Sutras*, the text on the philosophy of yoga believed to date back to the 2nd century BC. The first two limbs – the "Yama" and "Niyama" – can be seen as yoga "dos" and "don'ts". These are not laws, however, but rather guidelines for how you may want to construct your life. Some people choose to incorporate the principles of the sutras into their daily lives; others prefer not to. Do whatever is helpful to you.

Niyamas
Shauca – be pure
Samtosa – be content
Tapas – be disciplined
Svadhyaya – be studious
Isvara pranidhana – be devoted

Yamas
Ahimsa – do no harm
Satya – tell no lies
Asteya – do not steal
Brahmacharya – practise chastity
Aparigraha – don't be greedy

The benefits of yoga for mothers

You may feel many ups and downs during the early weeks after the birth – having a small person depend on you for everything brings both joys and challenges. Many women miss their independence and even feel that they have lost their own identity. Although you will cherish your baby, you may find the physical and emotional adjustments of new motherhood draining. Yoga will uplift you, restore you, and make you feel more positive about yourself and your role as a mother. It can be a support on days when you are low and on days when you are high – and most days you will feel a mixture of both!

It is quite common for women to feel somehow "disconnected" from their bodies during the early weeks after the birth. This book contains a gentle "Time for you" section (see pages 70–89), which will offer you guidance on how to integrate your body, mind, and breathing. The gentle exercises will relax your shoulders and upper back, releasing the tension that you may feel if you breast feed. The breathing exercises will refuel your energy and revitalize you when you are feeling tired.

Yoga is ideal for strengthening your pelvic floor in the early weeks after giving birth, using exercises that involve the movement known in yoga as "Mula Bandha", the contraction of the pelvic floor. The practice of "reverse breathing" (see page 72) draws your navel toward your spine as you exhale, tightening your abdominal muscles and toning your deep muscles. This is especially valuable if you have had a Caesarean section.

After giving birth you may feel weak overall, with tightness in your upper back and neck and pain in your lower back and pelvis. You may also suffer discomfort from an episiotomy, or tear. Gentle yoga practice, using asanas (postures and movements) applied correctly, will enable you to build up your strength and flexibility. Before starting any exercise programme, however, check with your physician.

HOW WILL YOGA HELP ME IF I'VE HAD A CAESAREAN BIRTH?
Your body may be feeling discomfort and restriction from the surgery of a Caesarean section. Although you will need to proceed gently, yoga will enable you to retrain your abdominal muscles, supporting and strengthening your lower back and abdominal wall. Reverse breathing and pelvic floor exercises (see pages 72–3) will promote recovery. You will be revitalized by breathing practices such as alternate nostril breathing (see page 73), which can facilitate relaxation after giving birth and aid with recovery after surgery. As your strength develops, you can progress to exercises for strengthening your abdominal muscles with the "Fly baby fly" sequence, alternate leg raises, and the "Mini boat" pose (see pages 52–3). But do not to start any of the exercises before you have checked with your physician.

HOW WILL YOGA HELP ME OVERCOME STRESS INCONTINENCE?
Your pelvic floor muscles, which line the pelvis from front to back and side to side, consist of separate layers that work together. During pregnancy and vaginal birth these muscles and their supporting ligaments can become stretched and weakened. This can lead to urinary incontinence in "stress" conditions, in other words when the muscles are under increased pressure, for example when you are coughing, laughing, or straining. Regular pelvic floor exercises (see page 73) can help to restore continence by

TIP You will need to practise pelvic floor exercises regularly before you will feel any change. If there is no improvement, or you are in discomfort, seek medical advice: there are other treatments available.

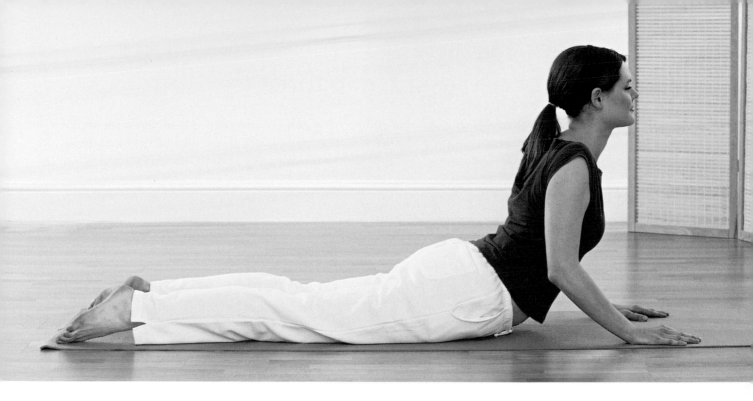

strengthening these muscle groups and are equally effective whether you practise them seated, semi-squatting, or lying flat.

WHAT IF I'M EXPERIENCING POSTNATAL DEPRESSION?

This condition, which is often under-recognized, can be caused by a combination of factors. Having a new baby carries with it many emotional demands: as a new mother, you will experience hormonal and physical changes, tiredness, and adjustments to your home life and family relationships. It is important to know that feeling low or "having the blues" is perfectly normal in the days after giving birth. Many women feel sad, irritable, tearful, tired, or even worthless at this time. It is only when the symptoms last for weeks or months and are more severe that we might describe a mother as having clinical depression. There is no shame or blame in feeling like this, so seek professional medical help if such symptoms continue.

Yoga, although it is not a "cure-all" remedy, can offer great support to other treatments for postnatal depression. Gentle physical exercise, such as that found within yoga, is a positive counter to depression. And practising yoga with your baby brings mutual

contact and interaction that will increase mother and baby bonding. The routines in this book will help you to release tensions and recharge your energy, leaving you with more to give to others and yourself.

Practising yoga with your baby will bring you pleasures from small and personal moments with your baby, such as mutual activity, togetherness, and smiles, and will give you "time out" to focus on each other. If you join a local baby yoga class in addition to practising at home with your baby, you will also benefit from the friendships and support networks that you will form with other mothers.

TIP Don't struggle alone if you feel low after having a baby. Many women "have the blues" at this time and networking with others may help you. Don't be afraid to seek professional medical help if necessary.

The benefits of yoga for babies

Baby yoga and baby massage can bring emotional and physical rewards for babies of all ages, and at each stage of development. As well as helping your baby to bond with you, it will soothe and stimulate her and help improve his balance, coordination, motor skills, and respiratory and digestive systems.

FROM 6 WEEKS TO 3 MONTHS

During your baby's first three months of life, her motor development will centre on gaining control of her head and neck muscles. She will hold her limbs close to her trunk at first and her hands in little fists. Her movements may appear a bit haphazard and she will be easily startled. Her vision will be rapidly improving and she will recognize her parents and other carers, gradually growing in trust, and will respond to facial gestures and pleasurable sensations.

At this stage, baby yoga provides visual stimulation, encouraging you and your baby to exchange facial expressions and body gestures. The exercises in the 6 weeks to 3 months section aid extension of the limbs through simple movements. Massage will encourage mutual trust and bonding through physical touch. It is important, however, not to embark on the following sequences before your baby has had her 6-week check. At this check up your medical practicioner will be able to assure you that you and your baby are ready to start the yoga exercises in this book.

FROM 3 MONTHS TO 6 MONTHS

From 3 to 6 months, your baby will be developing more complex movements and will be able to coordinate her muscle groups better. As her upper body control and strength develops, she will start to roll over. Her movements will be smoother and less jerky, her upper limb movements will become more directed and purposeful, and she will reach out to grab objects as her hand–eye control improves. Because she can now hold her head up and look around, she will be much more aware of her surroundings, including other people. As your baby's muscular control develops from her centre outward, she will be able to kick when lying on her back and lift his head and shoulders when lying on her tummy. She

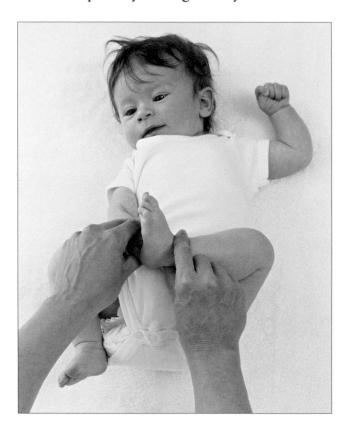

ABOVE Yoga exercises from 3 to 6 months can help your baby learn to control the movements of his individual limbs.

will start to roll over and maybe even sit up as his lower spine strengthens.

The routines for 3 to 6 months in this book make more use of active play, with fun routines, songs, and rhymes to encourage movement and social participation. As your baby attempts to learn to crawl, she will move individual limbs in a directed and coordinated way, and the exercises in this section use movements of each limb in turn, together with opposing leg and arm actions, to promote this.

How do I love thee? Let me count the ways.
I love thee to the depth and breadth and height
My soul can reach, when feeling out of sight....

Elizabeth Barrett Browning

Exercises with your baby lying on her tummy allow her to stretch her whole body and build up torso strength, while the rolling sequences allow her to exercise her whole body in fun routines. At this time she may be beginning to teethe, and the calming walks and "whooshing" sequences can help to relieve discomfort. Your baby will be more active socially and will enjoy the smiles and interactions that you share together in yoga. She will also enjoy watching your movements as you exercise.

FROM 6 MONTHS TO 9 MONTHS

At 6 to 9 months, your baby may be sitting up and will soon be starting to crawl. Babies use opposite arms and legs when crawling and this coordination will be helped by the yoga sequences. Many babies will be trying to stand at about 6 months and like to be supported in this position. They will be developing motor skills by reaching and grabbing things.

The exercises in this section are more interactive and playful, with song, rhymes, "peek-a-boo", and watching routines. Your baby will no longer wish to just lie on her back and will sit up to participate, so be prepared to adapt the exercises to her needs.

WHAT CAN I DO TO HELP MY PRE-TERM BABY?

Studies have shown that pre-term babies who are regularly stroked and regularly hear their parents' voices progress rapidly in early development. Pre-term infants who are massaged every day may cry less, go to sleep more easily, spend more time alert when awake, and show fewer signs of stress. Regularly massaged pre-term babies may also gain weight more quickly and will be more sociable and happy.

While your pre-term baby is still in hospital, you can use warm touch with relaxed hands as a daily routine. Once your baby is at home, you can begin to apply massage strokes to her, but respect when she has had enough. Hold her body in your cupped hands. To make sure that your hands are deeply relaxed as you do this, practise long, slow abdominal breathing (see page 18). You can use the massage routine in "Winding down" (see pages 66–9), but you will need to make a few modifications for a pre-term baby. Be sure that the space is very warm and that your baby is enclosed near you, then begin by massaging the place on your baby's body that has been least "invaded" when in hospital – this will usually be the back. Miniaturize every stroke – for example use two or three fingers rather than a whole hand. For more guidance, contact a qualified baby massage teacher (see the list of useful organizations on page 92).

HOW CAN I CALM MY COLICKY BABY?

A colicky baby will have difficulty in tolerating stimulation and will often be stiff and tense with a distended tummy. Babies with colic may gain a lot of comfort from the yoga sequences in this book, and the massage techniques can stimulate the gastrointestinal system and relieve colic. An effective relief routine for colic is the massaging the tummy sequence shown on page 67, followed by the "Knees to tummy" exercise on page 33. Many colicky babies also respond to relaxed holding – try the "soothing relaxed holding" and "calming walks with sounds" on pages 37 and 39 respectively. Remember that if your baby continues to be distressed she may be unwell, so seek professional medical help.

TIP By regularly massaging your baby you can help prevent, as well as alleviate, digestive problems.

The benefits of yoga for mothers and babies

Baby yoga will help you and your baby to get to know each other better. You will learn to interact with your infant in a more positive way and will begin to recognize his cues, which will enable you to provide the most appropriate care. This sort of "attunement" will give your baby the reassuring feeling of being emotionally connected to you and he will feel understood. As a mother, you will become more observant and will begin to notice your baby's unique qualities.

Baby yoga uses massage as a means for you to explore your baby. Touch is a positive way for you to get to know each other and has extensive benefits: you will develop a higher degree of mutual trust, your child will be less fractious and you will feel less anxious. You will communicate with your baby during massage as he watches you and you mirror his facial expressions. Through touch, you will learn to read "cues" such as changing expressions, yawns, and turning of the face or body. Understanding these cues will help you to interpret your baby's needs – for example is he tired or does he need a feed?

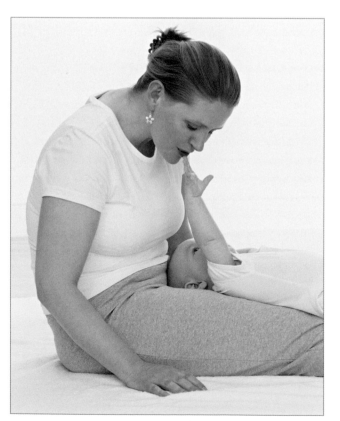

Touch will also have physical benefits for your baby. Studies have indicated that touch is important for a baby's healthy development, improving the function of the lungs, circulation, digestion, and hormone-secreting glands. In fact tactile stimulation can even contribute to the development of the infant brain and nervous system.

RECOGNIZING CRIES

Rather than feeding your baby as soon as he cries, try relaxed "whooshing" (see pages 39 and 54). Often your baby will just be tired or bored rather than hungry. Through baby yoga you can find ways of interpreting your baby's needs. Preventive routines and massage can help with colic, for example. Relaxation is also essential for you, the mother, so that you can cope calmly with testing times!

TIP If your baby cannot be comforted and is crying excessively, he may be ill. Do not attempt any baby yoga or yoga massage if he is limp and pale or has a temperature. Seek medical advice immediately.

PHYSICAL INTERACTION

How often do you just go up to your baby and tickle him for a smile? Yoga will help you to play and interact, promoting relaxation and helping your baby to sleep more deeply. Yoga routines consist of playing, stretching, and relaxation exercises with your baby,

LEFT Touch is important for your baby's physical and emotional wellbeing and will help the two of you to bond.

each of you focusing on the other. You will learn to handle your baby through movements and games that foster communication. He will receive positive body sensations, becoming relaxed and more able to deal with physical stress, and will enjoy the cumulative effects of touch, movement, rhythm, and relaxation. By focusing on your baby, you will understand how he communicates and you will grow in confidence through handling him and watching how he has fun – which can be fun for you too! Baby yoga fosters a rich non-verbal communication between mother and child, making happier mums and happier babies.

RELAXED BABIES MAKE RELAXED MUMS MAKE RELAXED BABIES

What can be better than taking time out to relax together? In practising the relaxation techniques in this book you will hold your baby close, providing reassurance and safety for her, as well as "letting go" emotionally and mentally. Yoga will help you to shift some attention away from your baby – yes, this is important too – putting your mind into neutral, sure in the confidence that your baby is looked after. Your baby will experience his mother free from superficial worry and will enjoy peace. You will see a pattern: when your baby relaxes, you will relax. And when both of you are relaxed, you will be better able to soothe and comfort your baby as well as yourself.

HELPING WITH SLEEP PROBLEMS

Every mother knows the desperation that comes when her baby will not go to sleep! Baby yoga can play a vital role in helping you cope with a wakeful baby by providing a firm routine of massage, which will allow your baby to relax and to sleep more soundly. This will help you to remain calm, which in turn will help your baby to feel secure, and the physical separation of bedtime will become less stressful for both of you. When your baby is sleeping better – and you, too, are getting more sleep – you will feel more able to meet his demands in a consistent and sensitive way.

SELF-AWARENESS

Yoga focuses on self-awareness and this is the key to empathy. By understanding our own emotions we can learn to read and recognize emotions in others. This can help us to remain in "neutral gear", maintaining balance and self-reflection even while our emotions are turbulent. This is a great help in parenting. Through relaxation in yoga you can learn to reflect on yourself and become aware of how your mood may affect your baby, and in this way you can avoid projecting your mood onto her. Breathing techniques will teach you to "centre" yourself in this way when you feel stressed – slow abdominal breathing (see page 17) will calm you down. Regular relaxation will help you to sleep and recuperate, which is very important when you have a young baby!

THE CYCLE OF JOY

Perhaps the main benefit of baby yoga is the fun and joy that you will share as mother and child. There is a cycle of joy, reciprocated and transferred from mother to baby and back again.

"When we laugh our heart rate goes up, our immune system is activated, hormones are pumped up to make us more alert and more oxygen flows to our brain, which seems to help us to think a bit sharper and see things more clearly. Our muscles relax and our digestive system works better. Stress levels go down. The air is less tense. We become capable of empathetic feeling, we become less hostile and our ability of making sound decisions and resolving conflicts improves." *Emotional Intelligent Parenting, Maurice Elias, Steven Tobias, & Brian Friedlander*

How to use this book

This book will guide you through massage and baby yoga sequences for babies from 6 weeks to 9 months old. Before you begin any sequence, make sure you have carefully read the important guidelines opposite on "When to practise and when not to practise". Then look at the "How to make your session more enjoyable" (see page 16), which will guide you through the practicalities of your session. You may need to refer back to this throughout your practice.

- At the beginning of each chapter, the "Getting started" recap will remind you how to begin a yoga or massage session with your baby.

- Make sure you work from the appropriate section of the book for your baby's age. You may need to be flexible about which exercises you try depending on his temperament. Allow your baby to guide you – some babies respond more to stimuli, while others prefer more gentle togetherness. Use your yoga session to observe your baby and learn what works well for both of you. You may find, for example, that your baby will want to do only one activity from the "To aid digestion" or "Play time" section. This is fine – by being receptive to his needs you will both benefit more from the session.

- The same guidelines apply to the "Time for you" section. Work in the appropriate timescale and never force your body. This may mean doing only a short relaxation session. Enjoy the small benefits – with time these will grow.

- Give yourself time to practise yoga every day, with and without your baby – but be patient with yourself. Your attitude will be crucial to any yoga that you do – remember that being a new mother isn't easy – there may be times when you feel frustrated and unhappy, or think you are a bad mother. Give yourself a break, realize that your feelings are normal, and ask for help if you need it. Let yoga accompany you as a friend and support during the exciting journey of motherhood!

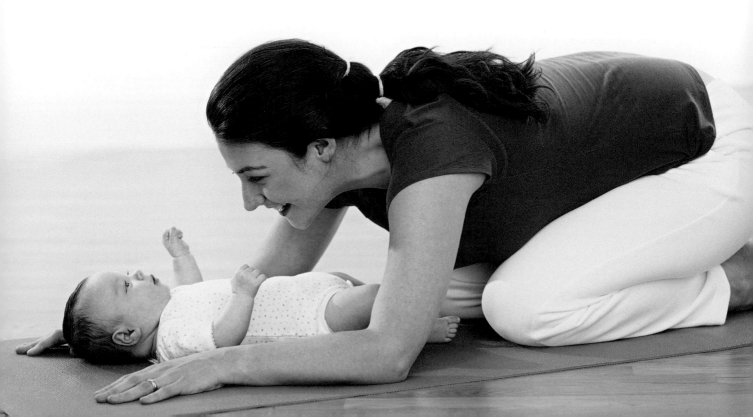

When to practise and when not to practise

Baby yoga provides an opportunity to experience fun and relaxation within a constructive framework. You and your baby will reap the rewards as long as you follow these simple guidelines to good practice.

DO

- Always follow similar routines – babies receive comfort from familiarity and enjoy recognizing patterns and predicting what will happen next.

- Always check you are comfortable and relaxed. Do a few warm-ups or breathing exercises yourself before you begin. This way you transfer only positive feelings to your baby.

- Always make sure your environment is calm and clean. The room should be warm and free from draughts with no light shining into your baby's eyes.

- Always work within the specific age limits given in this book and observe your baby's responses. Just because she wants an energetic practice today, it doesn't mean she will want the same tomorrow.

- Always focus on your breathing and posture throughout the practice. The more relaxed you are, the more relaxed your baby will be.

- Always use organic oils, such as sunflower, almond, sesame, grape seed or olive. Put a drop of oil on a small area of skin and leave it for 24 hours to see if your baby has a rash. Use alternative lubrication for a baby with eczema, following your doctor's advice.

- Always be aware of your own practice. Never force it, and be patient: it may take a while until you feel able to stretch to the extent you want to or are used to, but little by little you will experience benefit and improvement.

- Always include dads and siblings. Many older siblings enjoy massaging their own dolly and dads enjoy constructive play. Baby yoga is fun for everyone!

DON'T

- Do not undertake any of the yoga routines in this book until you and your baby have had your 6-week post-natal check up.

- Never practise on a distressed baby. If your baby gets upset, comfort her and stop the practice until she is calm.

- Never practise baby yoga if you feel angry. Leave the room for a few moments, take some deep breaths, or call a friend.

- Never use massage oils before doing energetic baby yoga as your baby may be slippery and you may drop him. Keep the oily massages separate from your play time in baby yoga.

- Never rush – choose a moment when you have time to spare and check the time is appropriate for your baby. Your baby won't want play time if she is hungry or tired.

- Never force any practice – if your baby doesn't like an exercise, stop and try again some other time.

- Never massage your baby or practise baby yoga directly after she has been immunized. Wait 48 hours as most babies will feel unwell.

- Never practise yoga with your baby if she is sick or unwell. If she has a fever, is limp, or has difficulties breathing, seek medical assistance immediately. If in doubt, call for help.

How to make your session more enjoyable

Creating a special yoga area, perhaps using a particular rug or blanket, is useful to tell your baby that yoga time has begun. Avoid a draughty room or one with bright sunshine and find a calm place where you won't be disturbed.

HOW DO I SIT? ▶

There are various ways to sit, but make sure you are comfortable – perhaps kneeling, or sitting cross-legged, with your baby on the floor in front of you. You can use a cushion to sit on or for leaning up against a wall if you need more support.

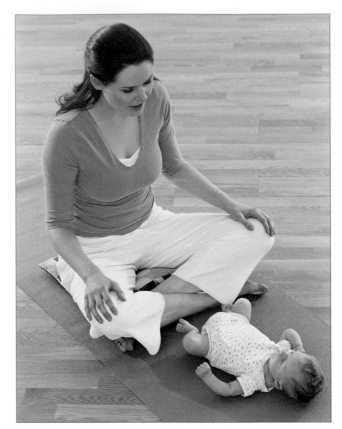

HOW DO I MAKE CONTACT? ▶

Involve your baby at the start of any session by asking her permission to proceed. At this time you can observe what mood she is in and what type of session (if any!) is best at this moment. You want to do yoga and massage with your baby, not to her.

Before you make contact, ask permission, gently saying "*Can I massage you?*", and wait for a positive response. If your baby isn't happy, comfort her and try again later.

1 Put your hands on your baby's body and gently massage her tummy in a clockwise motion.

2 It will be soothing and comforting for your baby if you hold her feet.

3 Give long massage strokes from the top of her body all the way down to her feet.

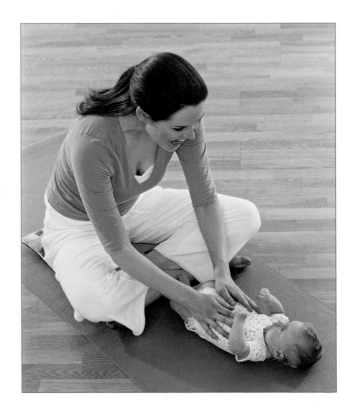

HOW CAN I RELAX? ▶

Try to "centre" yourself at the start of a session, using the following routine:

1 Sit comfortably and upright, focusing your mind on your breathing.

2 Put your hands on your chest and gently follow the pattern of your breathing, being aware of its rise and fall. Don't hurry, but concentrate on breathing slowly, allowing each breath to be fully exhaled before you inhale again.

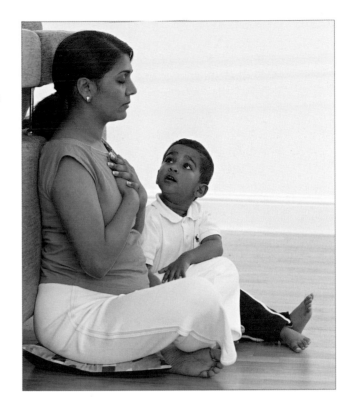

QUICK RELAXATION

This "quick relaxation" technique is a good one to try if you are worn out and need to recharge your batteries. You can try it with or without your baby.

1 Lie on your back on the floor with your feet turned outward and the back of your hands on the floor. Curl your fingers inward gently. Make sure that your neck is comfortable, with your head centred. Close your eyes and be aware of how you feel.

2 Concentrate on each part of your body in turn, starting with your feet and working upward through your lower legs, upper legs, hips and buttocks, then your hands, lower arms, upper arms, lower back, chest, shoulders, neck, and face. Each time you breathe out, focus on "letting go" and feel your body sinking back to the floor.

3 Now focus on your out breath: let it be a bit longer than your in breath, and count down from 10 as you slowly breathe out. Keep your breathing slow and unhurried. When you reach zero, slowly turn your head from side to side. Then, breathing in, stretch your arms up to the ceiling and above your head. As you breathe out, bring your arms back down to your side. Repeat this a couple of times.

When you are ready, turn onto one side of your body and slowly come back up to a sitting position.

BASIC YOGA BREATHING ▶

Relaxed breathing, which is integral to the practice of yoga, will help release tension and harmonize your mind and body, benefiting you physically, mentally, and emotionally.

1 Sit comfortably and place your hands on your chest. Be aware of your breath, and as you breathe in, feel your chest expand and your fingers rise up toward your head. As you breathe out, feel your chest and your fingers sink back down.

2 Place your hands on your rib cage. Feel your chest expand into your hands as you breathe in, then feel your hands fall back as you breathe out. Repeat this 3 times.

3 Bring your hands to your tummy. Breathe in and feel your tummy swell as you breathe in then subside as you breathe out. Focus on this movement.

4 Now combine all the above steps to make a full continuous flow of in and out breathing. This is the full yogic breath.

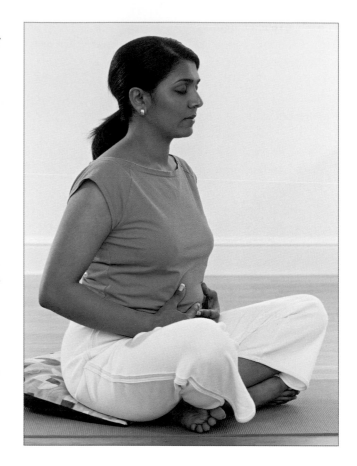

RELAXED HOLDING OF YOUR BABY

Throughout this book we talk about relaxed holding to comfort and soothe your baby. There are lots of ways in which you can do this, depending on your baby's age and mood. These are outlined below:

Basic face-down safety position, suitable from birth to 6 months

1 Make sure that your shoulders are relaxed. With your baby facing away from you, place your strong hand under his seat and between his legs to support his trunk. Support your baby's chest against your other arm.

2 Face your baby downward so that his head is aligned with his spine. Rest his head on your inner elbow, which will give it additional support.

Soothing, relaxed holding ▶

If your baby is very fretful, hold her against your body in the basic safety position described opposite, but this time facing outward.

1 Without moving your safety hand from between the legs, swivel your baby round sideways so that her spine stretches along your rib cage. If you are right-handed, her head should be to your left and vice versa.

2 Slide your seat hand up between your baby's legs so that it rests on her tummy. You can then gently massage her tummy as you walk around.

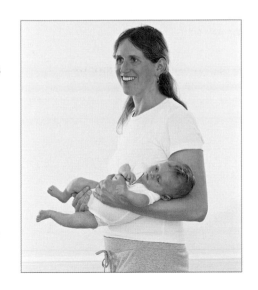

Upright holding ▶

Some babies are more soothed in an upright position.

1 Start with your baby in the seat-hold position described in step 1 on the opposite page.

2 Now bring him close to your body so that his head is resting on or just below your shoulder.

3 Use your weaker arm to support your baby's back while your strong arm remains under his seat.

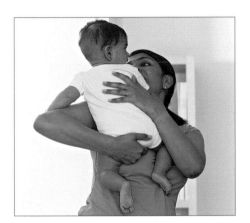

Relaxed holding on your hip, for the older baby from 6 months ▶

This is a variation of the basic safety position.

1 Sit your baby against your hip so that he is facing outward, and support him by placing your arm across his chest. You should be able to walk freely. Try to relax your shoulder and allow him to rest mainly on your hip bone.

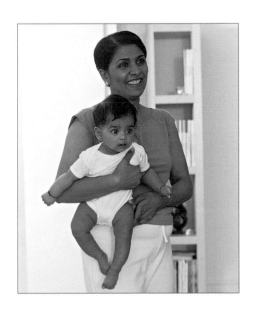

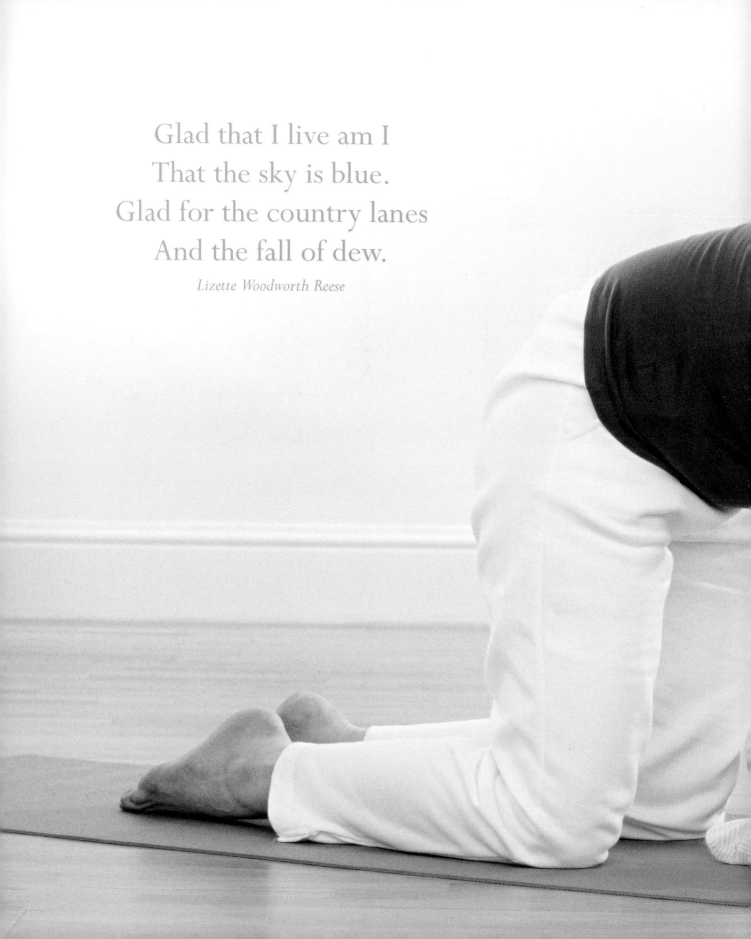

Glad that I live am I
That the sky is blue.
Glad for the country lanes
And the fall of dew.

Lizette Woodworth Reese

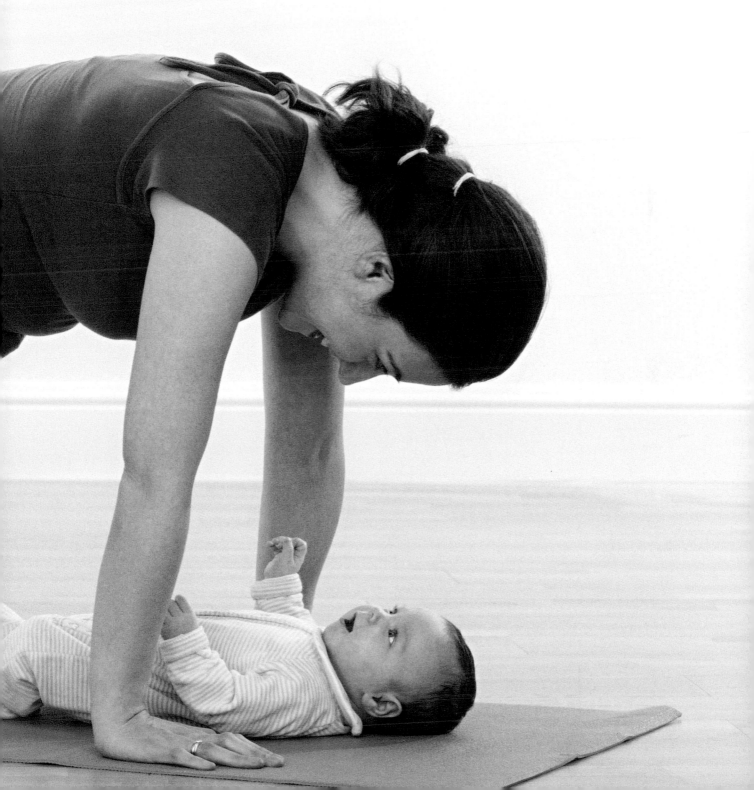

Warm-ups for mothers

Take a couple of moments to relax: "centre" yourself, release tension from your shoulders and back, and quieten your breathing. This way you will be ready to pass on only positive feelings to your baby.

Relaxing by "centring" ▶

Centring will help you balance your thoughts and quieten down before you begin your yoga practice.

1 Sit comfortably in an upright position and focus your mind on your breath.

2 Put your hands on your rib cage and gently follow your breathing, being aware of its rise and fall. Don't hurry: exhale each breath thoroughly before you inhale again.

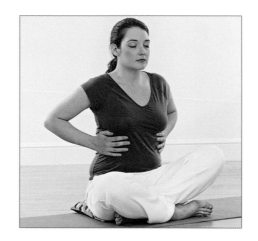

The prayer pose stretch ▼

This stretch will release tension from your upper back. It will also help you to slow down your breathing as you synchronize the movement with your breath.

1 Sit however you feel comfortable – this may be in a simple cross-legged position. Try to sit up as tall as you can. Begin by bringing your palms together in a prayer pose.

2 With your next in breath take your arms up above your head.

3 Then, as you breathe out, lower your arms down. Try to release your out breath with a long sigh.

Repeat this stretch sequence 4 to 6 times.

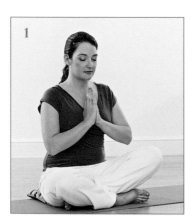
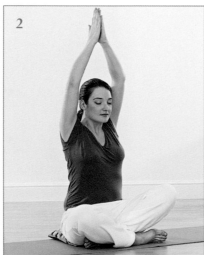
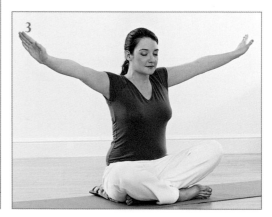

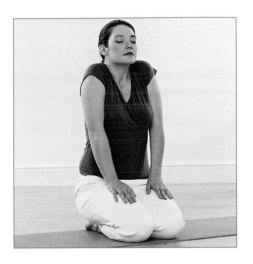

◄ Shoulder lifting

This exercise will help you release all the tension from your shoulders.

1 Sitting upright, with your hands on your knees, lift your shoulders to your ears as you slowly inhale.

2 Release your shoulders down as you breathe out.

Repeat this sequence 4 to 6 times.

Arm rotation ▼

1 Place your fingertips on your shoulders, with your elbows out in front of you. Try to keep your elbows as close together as possible.

2 While inhaling, lift your elbows up past your ears. As you breathe out, circle your elbows to the sides, then lower them down, dropping your shoulders.

Repeat the exercise 4 to 6 times.

TIP These exercises are wonderfully invigorating – you are undoing tension throughout your entire upper body. Do a few rounds and notice how you feel. Always remember to focus on your breathing.

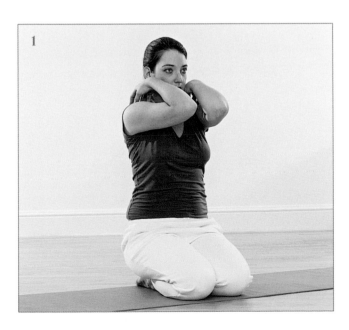

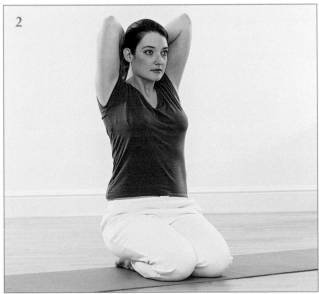

The cat pose ▶

This is a fine pose for releasing tension from your back. You can also enjoy it with your baby by placing him on the mat in between your hands and knees. Make it more fun for your baby by making cat noises as you look down at him in step 1!

1 Start the exercise by kneeling on the yoga mat in an all-fours position. Gently arch your upper back, tucking in your chin as you breathe out.

2 As you breathe in, bring your bottom up and look straight ahead so that your back straightens. Repeat this 4 to 6 times.

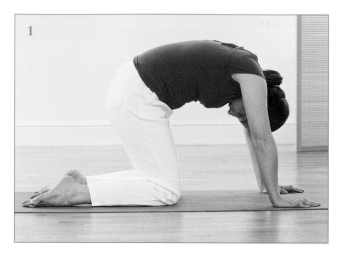

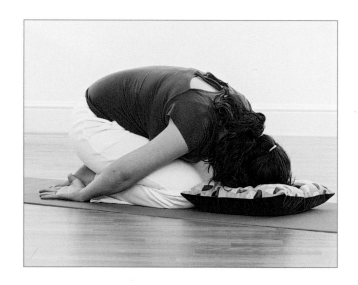

Child's pose ▶

This is a resting pose. Relax here for a few breaths before attempting the rolling cat (see opposite page).

1 Sit back on your heels, then bring your forehead to the floor. (Use a cushion to support your head if you wish.)

2 Rest your arms alongside your body with your palms facing up. The pose should feel completely relaxing. Breathe deeply and rest here for a few moments.

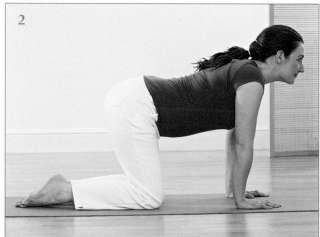

The rolling cat ▶

If you enjoyed the cat pose you can repeat it with a little more motion in this exercise. The rolling cat should consist of continuous flowing movements.

1 Starting from the same all-fours position as in the cat pose, tuck your bottom under and round your back, tucking your chin in as you breathe out.

2 As you breathe in, drop your bottom onto your heels and with your elbows on the ground, move your body forward so that you are rolling your nose across your baby's tummy.

3 When your shoulders are above your wrists, straighten your elbows, round your back, and tuck your chin under again to return to the beginning of the movement. This step should be done on the out breath.

4 Finally, rest in the child's pose (see opposite) for 3 long slow breaths.

TIP In yoga we try to breathe in through both nostrils and out through both nostrils. But if you are very tense you might find it beneficial to release a big "haaa" breath out of your mouth.

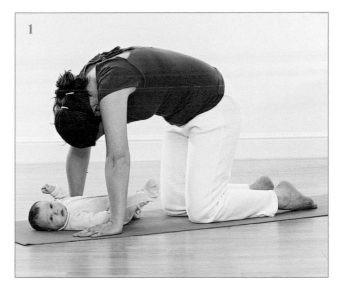

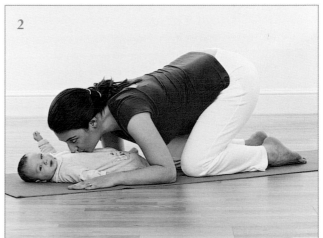

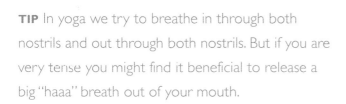

Warm-ups for babies

Warming up with your baby is essential. Not only does it prepare her for the yoga session ahead, it will allow you to observe your baby's mood and responses, which may sometimes mean adjusting your plans.

Making contact

1 Sit in a comfortable position with your baby lying down in front of you and facing toward you. Your baby can be fully dressed in comfortable clothes or wearing a vest, but make sure that her feet are bare.

2 Begin by thanking your baby for being patient and asking permission to start the practice. Ask *"Can I massage you?"*

3 If your baby seems happy, gently stroke her from the top of her body all the way down to her feet. Repeat this 2 to 3 times. Enjoy it and relax!

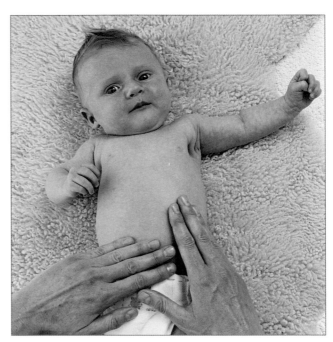

ABOVE Massage will encourage mutual trust and bonding between mother and baby through physical touch.

TIP As this is a warm-up and will be followed by baby yoga, don't use oils – you don't want to slip with your baby. If, however, you are only massaging your baby, feel free to use an oil, such as cold-pressed olive oil or sunflower oil. Make sure that you have tested the oil on a small patch of your baby's skin for 24 hours before using it for the first time, to check that he does not have an allergy to it.

Legs

An easy, enjoyable way to start massage and help your baby relax all over is with "Indian milking" of the legs.

1 Cupping the top of your baby's right leg in one hand, gently slide your hand down the leg. Repeat using one hand after the other.

2 Holding the leg in one hand just above the floor, gently drop it into your other hand. You can, if you wish, use this little rhyme to help your baby relax: *"Jiggedy jig, jiggedy jig, the farmer cuddled the pig. Relax, relax."* The leg should be nice and floppy.

3 Finish the leg massage with a long stroke from the top of the leg all the way down. Repeat this twice.

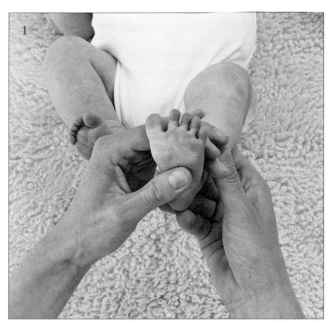

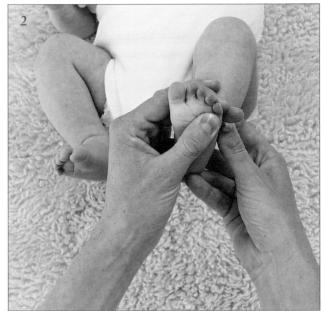

Feet ▲

1 With your thumb on the sole of your baby's right foot, gently massage the foot from the heel all the way up to the toes. Repeat this twice.

2 Gently press and then release the area under each of your baby's toes, one toe at a time, using your thumb. These are the reflexology points to help with teething pain.

3 Starting with his big toe, gently massage each of your baby's toes between your thumb and index finger. If you wish you can use the following rhyme:
Big toe – *"This little piggy went to market"*
Second toe – *"This little piggy stayed at home"*
Third toe – *"This little piggy had a massage"*
Fourth toe – *"This little piggy had none"*
Little toe – *"This little piggy went wee wee wee all the way home"*.
Then tickle your baby under the arms.

Repeat the whole leg and foot massage sequence on your baby's left leg and left foot. Don't hurry – enjoy the songs and the eye contact with your baby.

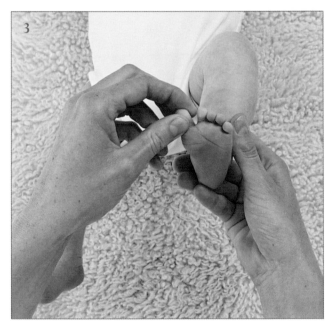

TIP Don't be embarrassed about singing to your baby – your voice may not sound fantastic to you, but to your baby it's perfect!

Chest ▶

Some babies love this massage, some don't. It can be very helpful if your baby is congested or has a cough.

1 Place both your hands on your baby's chest.

2 Move your hands gently in opposite directions to massage in little circles around the chest area with your fingers.

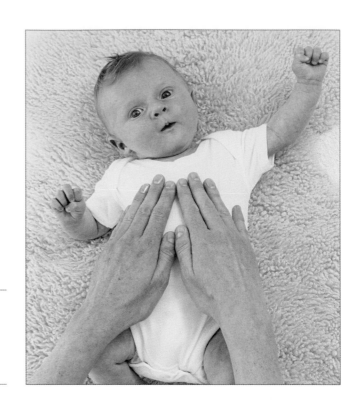

TIP Check your own posture. Sit tall and make sure that your neck and shoulders are relaxed. The more you relax, the more your baby will relax.

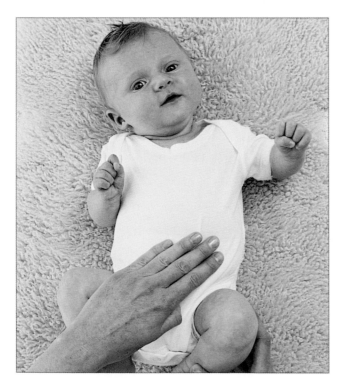

◀ Tummy

These massages are very helpful for wind pains or colic. Don't be surprised if your baby releases a bit of wind – this means it's working.

1 Move your hand down to your baby's abdomen and, using your fingers, gently massage in a circle clockwise to follow your baby's digestive tract. Your baby's abdomen should feel soft and spongy not hard.

2 Be careful not to press too hard on your baby's abdomen as she will not like this. You can sing the nursery rhyme "Round and round the garden" or another of your baby's favourite songs if you wish.

The arms ▶

For this massage, your baby can either remain lying on a rug in front of you or, if she is restless, you can sit her up on your lap.

1 Begin with "Indian milking", cupping your baby's arm in your hand and sliding your hand from the top of her arm down to his wrist. Continue using one hand after the other. Sing a song if you wish.

2 Relax the whole arm by gently dropping it into your other hand. Sing *"relax, relax"*.

3 Use long strokes all the way down the arm to finish the arm massage.

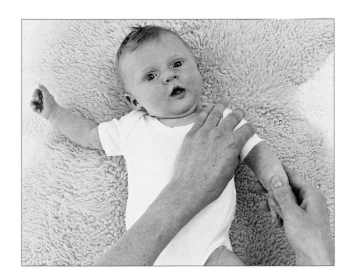

Hands and fingers ▼

1 Encourage your baby to keep her hands open and gently massage her palm using your thumb.

2 Gently massage each of his fingers, one at a time, singing *"This little piggy"* as in the toe massage (see page 27, step 3).

3 Gently drop the arm, then stroke from the top of the arm all the way down (see steps 2 and 3 above).

Repeat all the arm, hand, and finger massages slowly on the other arm. You can sing as many songs as you wish while doing so!

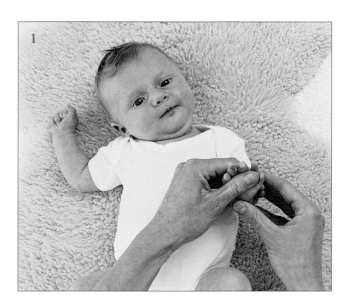

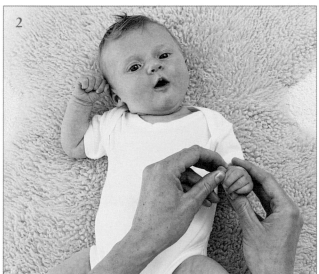

My babe is so beautiful!
It thrills my heart with tender gladness,
Thus to look at thee.

Samuel Taylor Coleridge

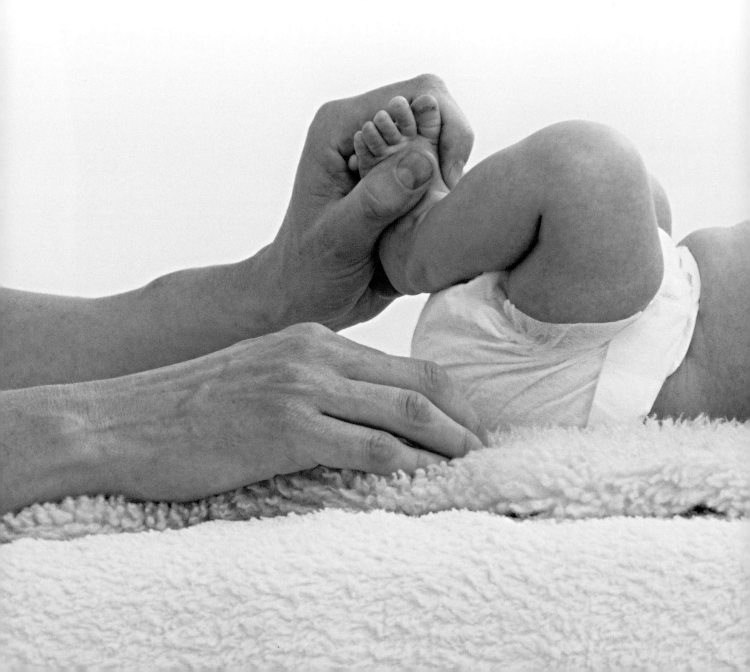

Exercises:
from 6 weeks to 3 months

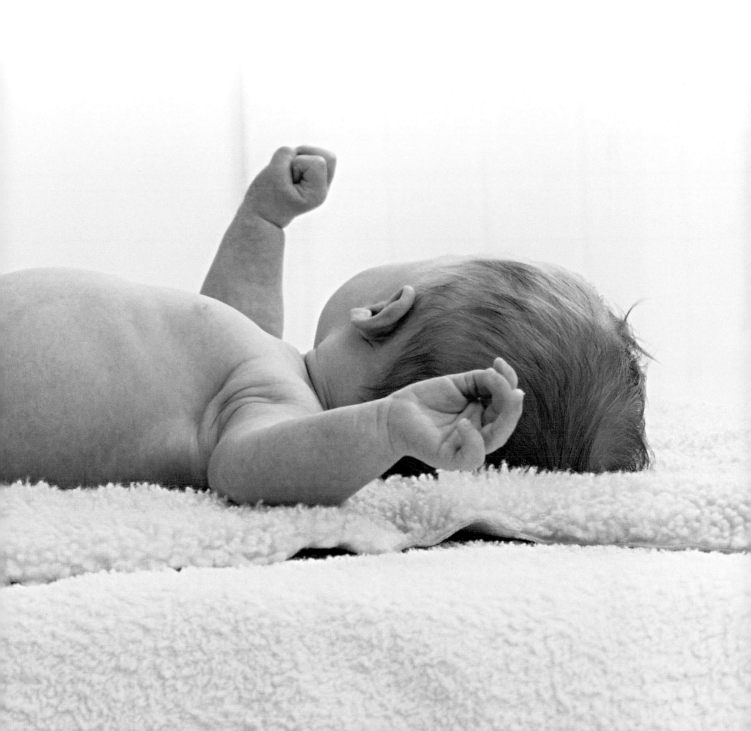

From 6 weeks to 3 months

Your baby's main developmental needs at this time are to bond with you, develop her vision, and master her head and neck control. Her attention span may be short, so watch for when she's had enough. You may find that at the start she won't complete a whole routine – just try one or two exercises and stop when she needs to. With time you can build up the sequence.

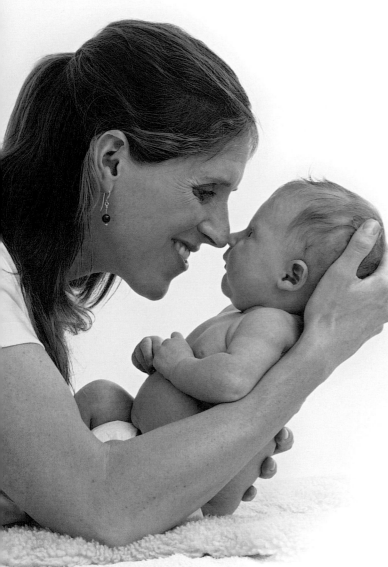

GETTING STARTED – a recap

1 Relax – centre yourself and do a few stretches.

2 Create a setting.

3 Check your position.

4 Make contact.

5 Begin with a warm-up followed by the appropriate sequence for your baby's age and mood.

Waking-up time

Making contact – see page 26

Gentle dry massage – see pages 26–9

To aid digestion

The following sequence introduces exercises to help your baby's digestion. Wind pains and colic are quite common at this stage of a baby's development. You can do these poses with your baby on your yoga mat in front of you or, if you prefer, with her lying on your lap.

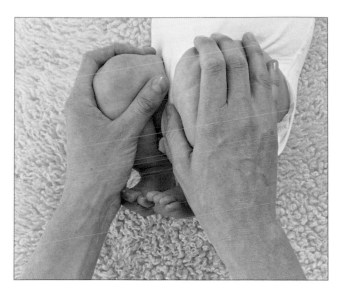

◄ Knees to chest

1 Sit in a comfortable position, such as a simple cross-legged pose.

2 Place your hands on your baby's knees and breathe in. As you breathe out gently bring your baby's knees toward her tummy.

Repeat this movement a few times.

TIP This pose stimulates the digestive system and may produce a burp or bowel movement.

Knees from side to side

1 With your hands in the same position as before, bring the bent knees of your baby together in alignment and move them over to the left and then to the right.

2 Repeat this a few times.

TIP This posture works as a gentle twist.

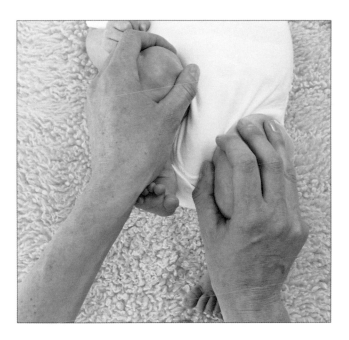

◄ Single knees to tummy

1 Place your hands on your baby's knees and gently bring one knee at a time to her tummy in a slow pedalling action.

2 Repeat this a few times.

TIP Never force this – or any other – movement. If your baby doesn't like this exercise, stop.

Hip circles ▼

1 Place your hands on your baby's knees and breathe in. As you breathe out gently bring your baby's knees toward her abdomen.

2 With your hands still on your baby's knees, gently trace a circle with the knees, rolling them in one direction and then the other. Repeat a few times.

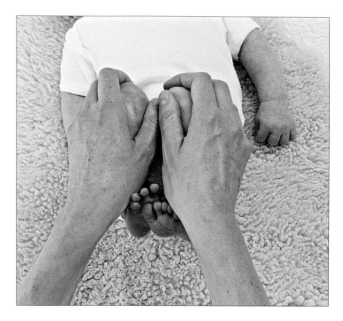

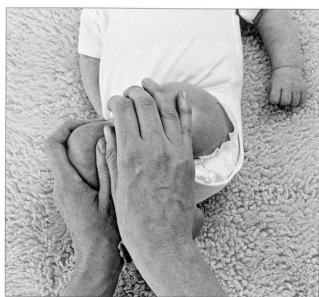

Mini lotus ▶

This exercise will increase your baby's suppleness and tone the muscles in the abdomen and back.

1 Gently take your baby's right leg and place it into the left inner thigh, without forcing it. Gently stroke the leg that you have moved.

2 Release the leg and repeat the exercise on the other leg.

TIP Never force this – or any other – movement. Stop at once it if your baby doesn't like it.

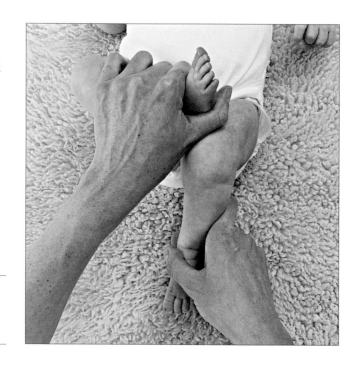

Butterfly ▼

This posture increases flexibility in your baby's hips.

1 Hold your baby's ankles in one hand and bring the soles of the feet together.

2 Gently push the feet toward the tummy.

3 Release the pose and then repeat 2 or 3 times.

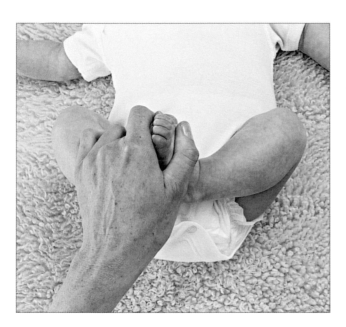

Butterfly circles ▼

1 Bring the soles of your baby's feet together in one hand and move them toward the tummy as before.

2 Gently move the legs in a circle in one direction and then the other.

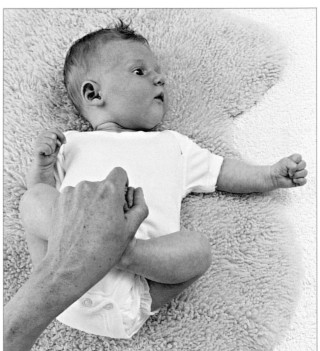

Leg stretch and drop

This posture shows your baby the difference between stretching and relaxing. You can make it fun by saying *"Up and down"* or *"Up and let go"*.

1 Hold your baby's ankles and lift her legs up slightly, extending them a little, then gently drop them down.

2 Repeat this a few times.

TIP At this age your baby's legs are naturally bent – they look a little like frogs' legs. You may not wish to stretch your baby's legs so do not force this – or any other – movement if you are not comfortable with it.

Arms open and close ▼

1 With your baby lying on her back in front of you, gently hold her arms together at the wrists and stretch her arms open as you inhale.

2 As you exhale, bring her arms back together again. You can make this more fun by saying *"open... open...open...close...close... close"*.

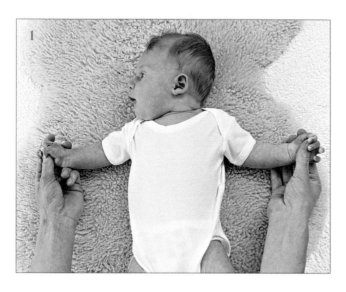

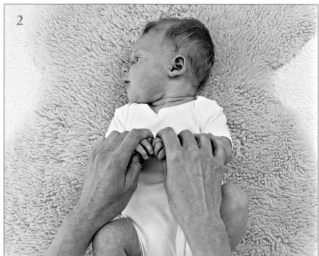

Arms cross and stretch ▼

If your baby is comfortable with the previous exercise, try this one.

1 Inhale and gently cross your baby's arms, without forcing, as if she is giving herself a big hug.

2 As you exhale stretch her arms open.

You can make this more fun by saying *"big hug"* as your baby crosses her arms and *"big stretch"* as she opens her arms wide.

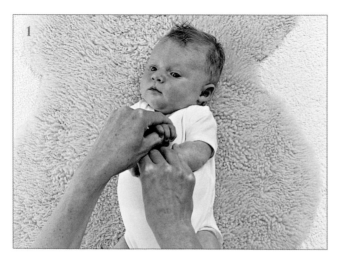

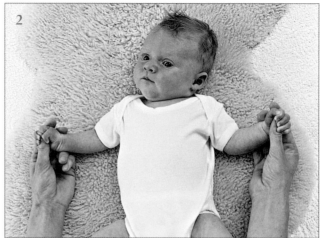

Grizzly time

There are times when your baby becomes "grizzly". This can feel very difficult and trying, and often happens just when you feel tired and less able to cope. Many young babies have colic and others just can't settle. Try the following routine to soothe her, and don't forget to take long slow breaths yourself.

Soothing relaxed holding ▶

1 Facing your baby away from you, place your strongest hand under her seat and the other hand across her chest.

2 Without moving your safety hand, swivel your baby sideways so that her spine stretches along your rib cage.

3 Slide your seat hand between your baby's legs so that it rests on her stomach and gently massage her stomach as you walk around.

4 Take long slow breaths.

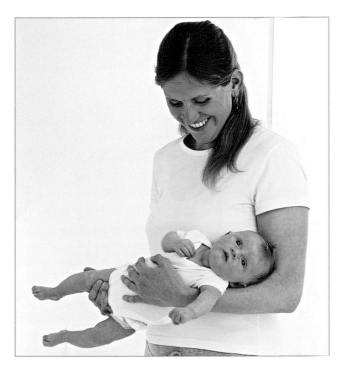

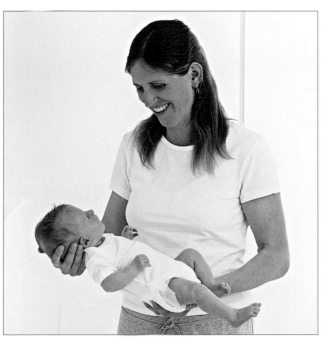

◀ Cradling seat hold

1 Use your strongest hand as a base under your baby's bottom to make a seat.

2 Support her head with your other hand, making sure that you also support the base of her neck.

3 Gently rock your baby from side to side.

Grizzly time checklist

If your baby is very grizzly, check that none of the following reasons are causing her discomfort.

- Is she hungry?
- Does she need a nappy change?
- Is she too hot or too cold?
- Is she unwell?
- Does she have wind?
- Is she bored?

Some babies, however, respond more to movement and action when they are grizzly, especially if they are just bored. If the soothing relaxed holding doesn't help, try some more gentle "action" yoga sequences. The sequence below should help if your baby has a tummy ache or if she is bored.

TIP Remember to sing to your baby! You may not feel like singing but the more you do, the more endorphins you produce, and the happier you will feel. The happier you are, the happier your baby will be. Any song will do.

Mini drops ▶

This can be an effective way to soothe a young and fractious baby. This sequence will not help if your baby is hungry, needs changing, or is unwell.

1 With your baby facing away from you, place one hand under her seat and your other arm across her chest to support her.

2 Gently lift her up with your seat hand and then let your arm drop a little, while continuing to hold her in the same way.

3 Repeat this a couple of times if your baby enjoys it.

TIP Make sure that you move slowly with no shaking, jerky movements and that you provide full support for your baby's neck and head with your arm across her chest.

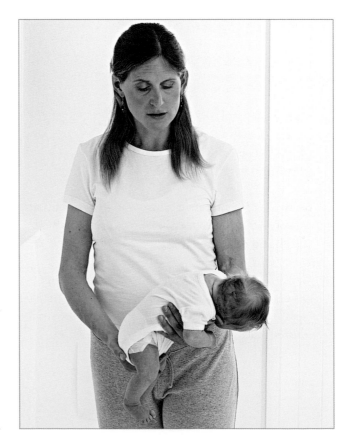

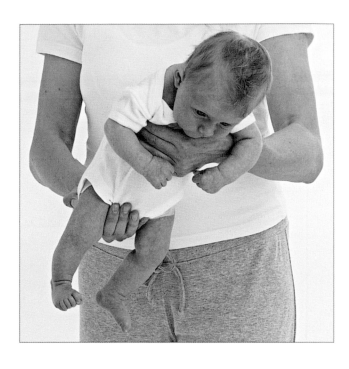

◄ Mini whooshes

1 Hold your baby in the same position as for the mini drops opposite, with one hand under her chest and your strong hand under her seat.

2 Gently swing your baby from side to side. You can increase the movement if she seems to be enjoying it.

TIP Mini whooshes can be an effective way to soothe a fretful baby, but never continue if she is distressed and not responding.

Calming walks with sounds ►

1 Hold your baby in the soothing relaxed hold shown on page 37.

2 Start gently walking, being aware of your breath. Exhale to help release any tension, doing so a few times if necessary. Then try to deepen your in breath and lengthen your out breath.

3 Be aware of your baby against you – with you, but separate. Walk in rhythm, being aware of each in breath and each out breath.

4 Gently start making the sound "*om*" on each out breath. (The sound will be more like a long "*Ahh oh hmmm*".) As your tension begins to disappear, your relaxed state will help to calm your baby, too.

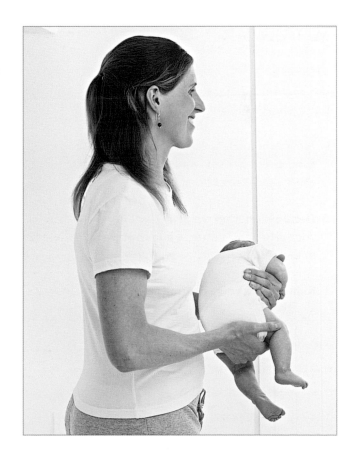

My heart is like an apple-tree
Whose boughs are bent with thick-set fruit....
My heart is gladder than all these,
Because my love is come to me.

Christina Rossetti

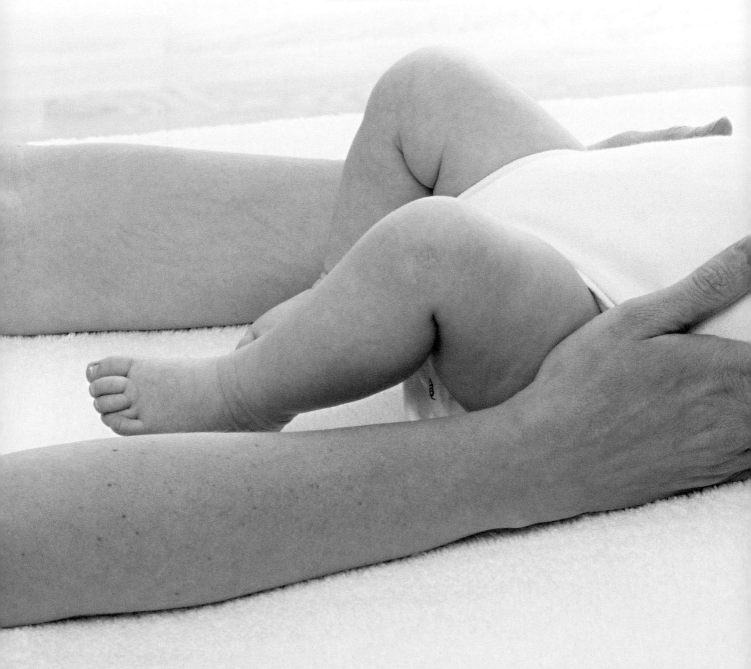

Exercises:
from 3 months to 6 months

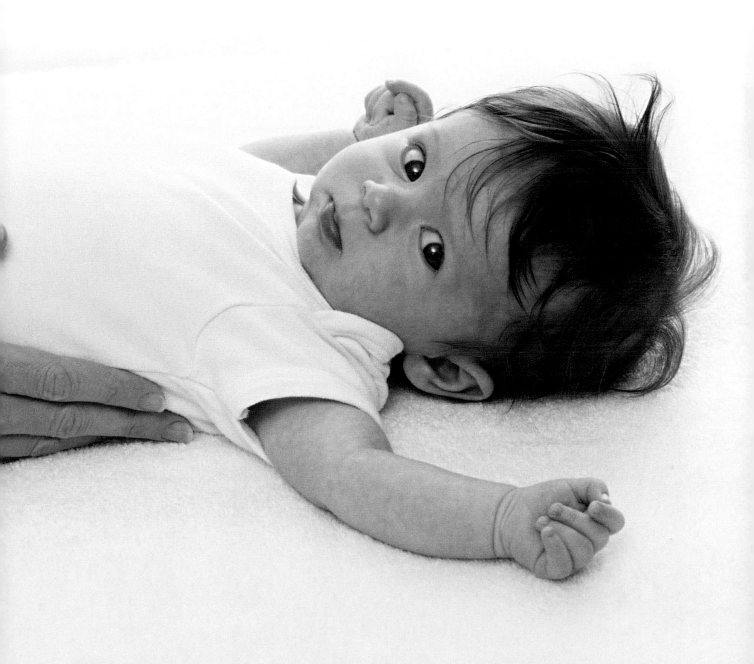

From 3 months to 6 months

Your baby will now be starting to make more complex coordinated movements. She will gain upper body strength and control and may roll over. The exercises in this section are slightly more energetic than those in the previous section but, as earlier, you should still follow your baby for guidance. As she will be more social now, why not meet up with a friend and do baby yoga with your children together?

GETTING STARTED – a recap

1 Relax – centre yourself and do a few stretches.

2 Create a setting.

3 Check your position.

4 Make contact.

5 Begin with a warm-up followed by the appropriate sequence for your baby's age and mood.

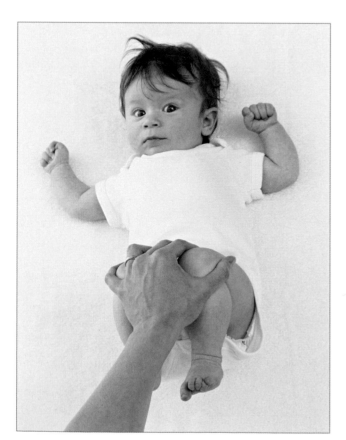

Waking-up time

Making contact – see page 26

Gentle dry massage – see pages 26–9

Hip sequence to aid digestion

This exercises below are similar to those for babies from 6 weeks to 3 months but can be made more energetic. Sing some of your favourite songs to accompany the movements!

◄ **Hip circles**

1 Place your hands on your baby's knees and gently roll the knees in one direction.

2 Now roll the knees in the other direction. You can make sounds to make it more fun, or say "one way" and the "other way".

Single knees to tummy

1 With one hand still on your baby's knee, gently bring one knee at a time to his abdomen.

2 Repeat this a few times, adding some rhythm to the movements.

TIP Be careful not to force these movements.

Half lotus ▼

1 Gently bring your baby's right foot toward her left upper thigh.

2 Now bring her left foot to the right inner thigh and release. Repeat this a few times, making it energetic and fun and saying *"criss cross, criss cross"*.

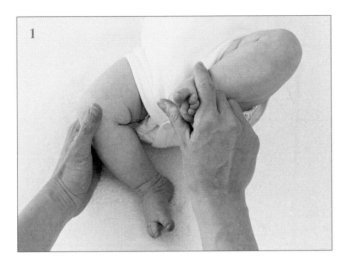

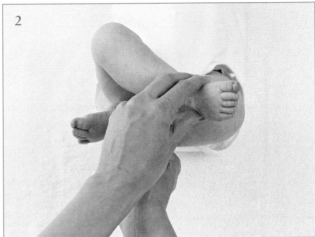

Spinal twist with massage ▼

This gentle twisting exercise will strengthen your baby's whole spine and help to open out his chest and shoulders.

1 Still lying on her back, hold your baby's bent knees together over her tummy with your left hand.

2 Breathe out and bring his knees over to your left in a straight line. At the same time, massage his left shoulder gently with a light movement.

3 Repeat on the other side, then allow her legs to relax and drop into your hands. Say "relax, relax".

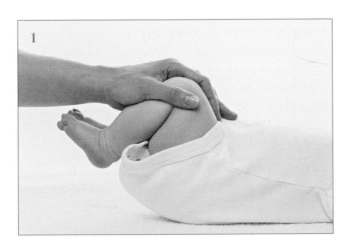

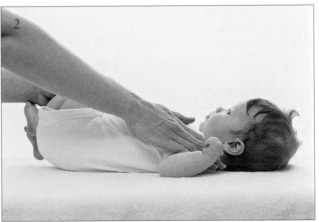

Exercises: from 3 months to 6 months 43

Diagonal stretch ▶

This exercise provides a counterpose to the spinal twist. Make it fun but never force the stretch.

1 Take hold of your baby's right foot and left hand and bring them together.

2 Open the arm and leg out again diagonally, then repeat with the left foot and right hand.

3 Repeat the whole exercise, this time saying *"Bind, bind, bind, bind"* when you bring your baby's foot and hand together and *"Big stretch, stretch, stretch, stretch"* when you stretch out the arm and leg.

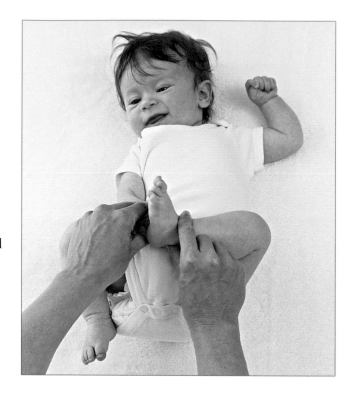

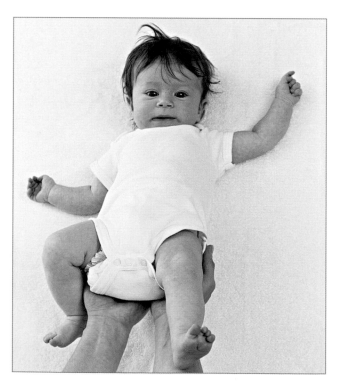

◀ Leg lifts and drops

This sequence ends with a relaxing posture.

1 Gently place your hands under your baby's bottom and lift his hips up.

2 Slide your baby down as you release his legs to the floor. You can add rhythm to the movement and say *"Up and drop"*.

3 Repeat the exercise a few times.

TIP Take care that the back of your baby's neck and head stay on the floor during this exercise.

Butterfly

1 Gently take your baby's right foot toward the left inner thigh. Do not force this movement and stop if your baby doesn't like it. Then take the left foot toward the right inner thigh.

2 Bring the soles of your baby's feet together without forcing it. Holding the ankles, push both legs gently toward the baby's abdomen.

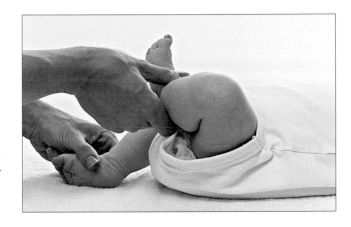

TIP At this age you can introduce some rhythm by pushing the feet twice toward your baby's abdomen then clapping them together.

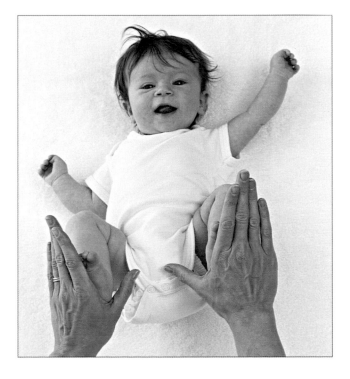

Push and counter push

1 Gently but firmly press the palms of your hands against the soles of your baby's feet.

2 Release and repeat a few times. With time, your baby will resist and push against your hands.

TIP When you feel your baby responding by pushing against your hand you can push a little harder. Make it fun. Try saying *"push...push... push...let go...push...push...push...let go"*. Your baby will enjoy the challenge.

Play time

Your baby is now a little older and will enjoy sitting on your lap and watching other adults or babies. Try the following arm exercises and make them fun and energetic.

Arm and chest opening, from sitting

As your baby becomes more confident she will be able to increase how much she can stretch and therefore breathe more deeply. This is the essence of yoga.

1 Sit your baby on your lap with her back to you. Hold onto her hands and gently open her arms wide.

2 Bring her hands back together again. Be careful not to force either movement.

3 Repeat this exercise a few times. You can introduce rhythm into the movements and say "*open…open… open*" and "*close…close…close*".

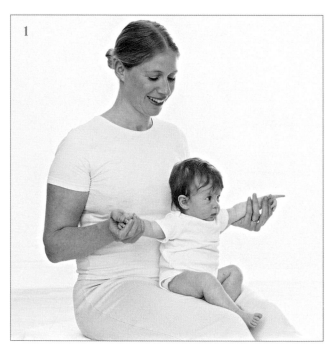

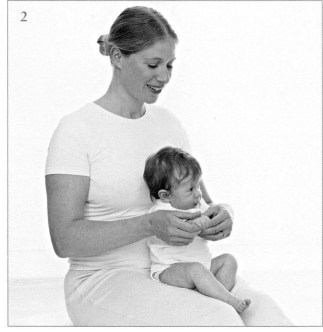

Windscreen wipers

This movement introduces a song and accompanying actions to vary the arm stretches.

1 With your baby still sitting on your lap, bring her hands together and open them up again as in the arm and chest opening exercise above. This time

when your baby closes her arms she's giving herself a big hug

2 Next try the exercise with the following song: "*Windscreen wipers, windscreen wipers, what do you do all day? Swish… swosh…swish…swosh… we wash the rain away*". Do the actions as you sing the song.

Wind and punch ▾

1 With your baby still on your lap, gently hold her hands and start winding them in a circular action. Say "*wind…wind…wind…wind*".

2 Still holding onto your baby's hands, stretch one of her arms forward as if in a little punching movement with one hand and say "*punch*".

3 Put steps 1 and 2 together, saying "*wind…wind… wind…wind…punch*". Repeat a few times.

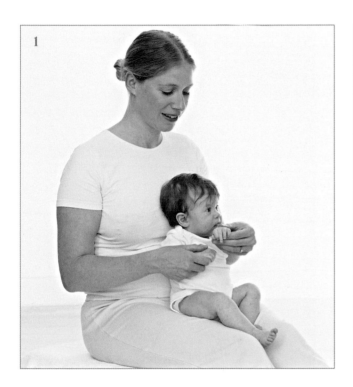

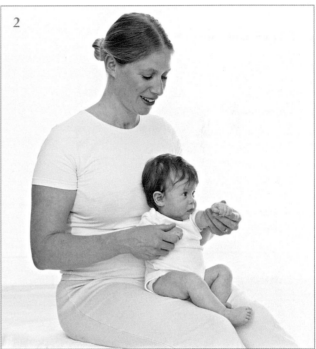

Wind the bobbin up

This is another action song that you can do with your baby sitting on your lap. Hold her hands and guide him through the movements:

"*Wind the bobbin up*
Wind the bobbin up (with a winding movement)
Pull…pull (pull arms open)
Clap…clap…clap! (hands together to clap).

(repeat the above)

Point to the ceiling (one hand up)
Point to the floor (one hand down)
Point to the window (one hand right)
Point to the door (one hand left).

Wind the bobbin up (with a winding movement)
Wind the bobbin up
Pull…pull (pull arms open)
Clap…clap…clap! (hands together to clap).

Back stretches

The following routines will help strengthen your baby's back muscles in preparation for crawling. They will also stimulate the digestive system and develop her breathing. For the back stretches, sit with your legs out in front of you with a straight upright back. You can sit on a cushion if this is more comfortable.

TIP You may find that you feel more secure if you sit on a duvet or have cushions near you.

Roller coaster ▼

1 Lay your baby on her tummy across your extended legs. Make sure she is comfortable and well supported by holding her ankles with one hand and placing your other hand on her upper back.

2 Gently lift up your leg under your baby's lower body so that her head is lower than her feet.

3 Now lower this leg and lift your other leg so that your baby's chest is higher than his bottom. Make the movement rhythmical like a see-saw, but check that your baby is well supported throughout.

4 Repeat, increasing the movement by lifting your leg up a little higher if your baby is enjoying it.

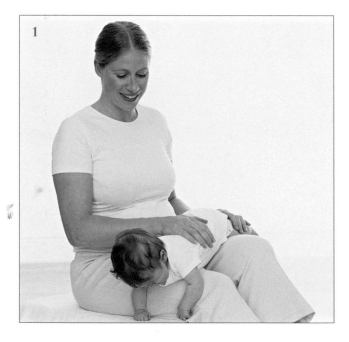

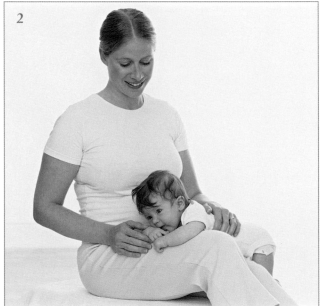

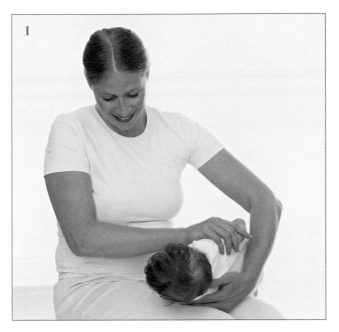

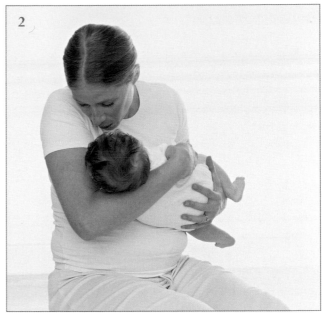

Rolls

These rolls will prepare your baby for crawling and will give her a chance to stretch her whole body and show independence in a fun way.

1 Lie your baby on her tummy across your legs, gently tuck in her arms, and roll her down your legs.

2 When you have rolled her to your knees, roll her all the way back up and give her a big kiss.

TIP Adapt this movement for your baby's taste and ability. If she doesn't like it, stop and cuddle her.

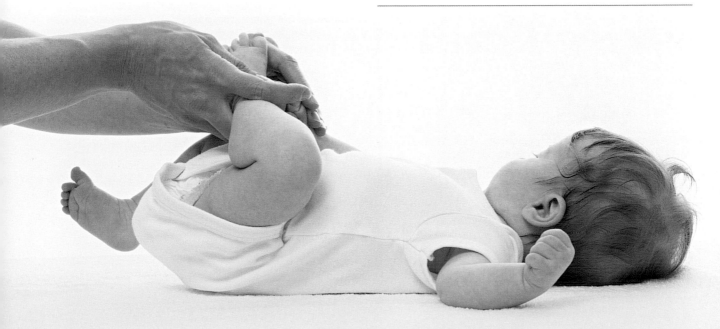

See-saw balances ▶

Many traditional yoga postures involve balancing, which not only stretches the legs and back muscles but also improves "centering" of the mind and body. Your baby's nervous system will also benefit from these gentle exercises.

1 Sitting with your legs out in front of you, sit your baby on your lap, facing to the side. Support her chest with one arm and provide support for the back of her head by placing your other hand on her upper back.

2 Create a see-saw movement, gently rocking your baby backward and forward.

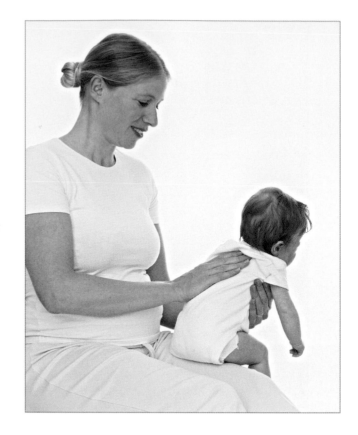

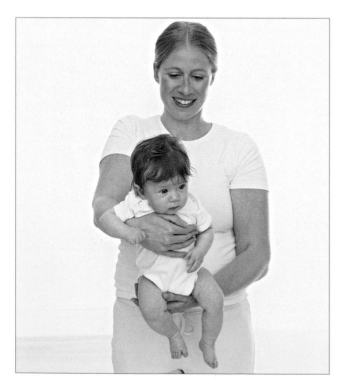

Seat balances ◀

This is a slightly more advanced exercise than the previous one. This pose will encourage your baby to strengthen her spine. You may want to do this exercise sitting on the bed or on a duvet on the floor for safety.

1 Support your baby with one hand under her bottom like a seat and your other arm making a "banister" support in front of her chest.

2 If you and your baby feel comfortable, release your arm from the front of your baby's chest for a few seconds, allowing him to balance on your seat hand.

3 Repeat this movement a few times.

Seat drops

This is a more energetic version of the mini drops (see page 38). If seat drops seem too much for your baby, go back to doing the mini drops for a while.

1 From standing, hold your baby with your strong hand under her seat and the other across her chest to support her. Keep your baby's back to your chest so she is looking forward.

2 Holding your baby with the same hold, breathe in deeply. As you breathe out, bend your knees in a little jerky movement, allowing your body to feel the little drop as you bend your knees. Do this a few times. Begin very gently and if your baby enjoys it, make it more energetic.

Try this song – when the frog says "croak", bend your knees allowing a little drop.

I'm a little frog and I say	– standing up
Croak...croak...	bend knees
I'm a little frog and I say	– standing up
Croak...croak...croak...	– alternate bending your
Croak...croak...croak...	knees with little drops
	at each croak

Lift-ups ▶

These gentle lift-ups will work your arm muscles as well as provide entertainment for your baby.

1 Sit in an upright comfortable position with your baby on your lap and place your hands under his armpits.

2 Inhale and gently lift her up, then exhale and bring him down.

3 Repeat this a couple of times.

TIP Try these exercises in front of the mirror. Your baby will find it very amusing to see herself as you sing this song.

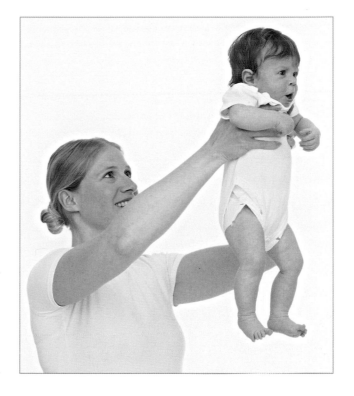

Lying down

The following postures are a fun way of doing a bit of yoga for yourself, working your abdominal muscles, while involving your baby. Exercise gently and stop immediately if you experience any pain.

Mini bridge ▶

This is a good exercise to work on – it knits together the abdominal muscles and tones the back of the legs.

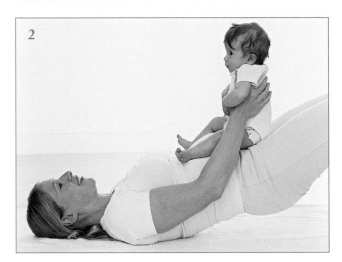

1 Lie down on your back with your knees bent. Sit your baby on your pelvis with her back resting against your thighs and support her position by placing your hands under her armpits.

2 As you breathe in, gently lift up your pelvis, keeping your shoulders on the floor. Lower to the ground as you breathe out. Repeat this a few times.

3 You can combine this movement with exercising your pelvic floor muscles. Breathe in, gently raise your pelvis, and draw in your pelvic floor. Breathe out, lower your pelvis, and release your pelvic floor.

Alternate leg raises ▶

1 Lie on your mat with your legs bent. Rest your baby against your thighs and support her as in the previous exercise.

2 As you breathe in, straighten one leg and gently extend it up into the air, keeping the other leg bent. Point your heel toward the ceiling.

3 On your next out breath, gently lower the extended leg down to the ground. Repeat this exercise several times with each leg.

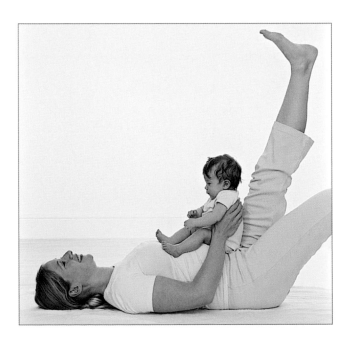

TIP If this exercise causes any pain stop at once.

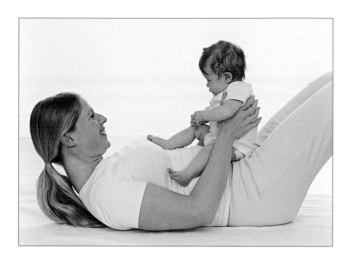

TIP It is important to avoid straining your neck so don't hold this pose. Lift your head gently – remember to keep breathing – and release smoothly.

◄ Mini boat

You need abdominal strength for this pose; if it feels too testing come back to it another time.

1 Lie on the floor and bend your knees, keeping both feet on the floor. Sit your baby on your pelvis, making sure that he is well supported as before.

2 Breathe in and gently lift your head and shoulders off the ground. Focus on drawing your navel to the base of your spine while you look up at your baby.

3 As you breathe out, gently release your head and shoulders back down to the ground.

4 Repeat this as many times as feels comfortable.

Fly baby fly ►

This exercise works on your abdominal muscles and allows your baby to have fun while watching you. Do not try this sequence when your baby has just eaten.

1 Lie on your back, holding your baby on your tummy. Lift your legs up with your knees bent. Bring your knees toward you and place your baby facing you on your shins. Keep her well supported.

2 Holding your baby securely on your shins, bring your knees toward you, gently drawing your tummy toward your spine, as you breathe in. Breathe out as you move your knees away from you. Repeat as many times as feels comfortable.

3 Checking that your baby is secure, lift her off your legs and bring your legs down to the floor. Place her on your tummy and relax.

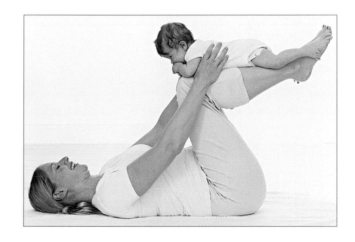

TIP If you have problems lifting your baby up on to your shins, ask someone to help you.

Grizzly time

If your baby suffered from colic it should be improving by this age, but she may now be beginning to teethe, which can bring new challenges for you in comforting her. The following sequences may help.

Soothing relaxed holding ▶

1 Place your stronger arm across your baby's chest and support her seat with your other hand.

2 Without moving your safety hand from between her legs, swivel your baby sideways so that her spine stretches along your rib cage and most of her weight is supported by your arm under her chest.

3 Slide your seat hand between her legs so that it rests on her stomach and massage her stomach as you walk around. Breathe long slow breaths.

TIP If your baby does not yet have full head control, rest your baby's head into your inner elbow.

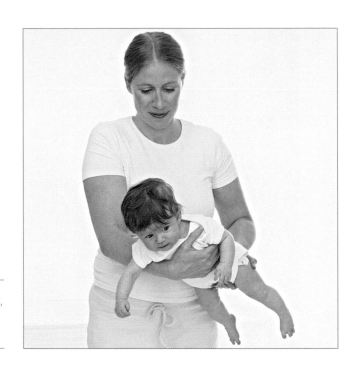

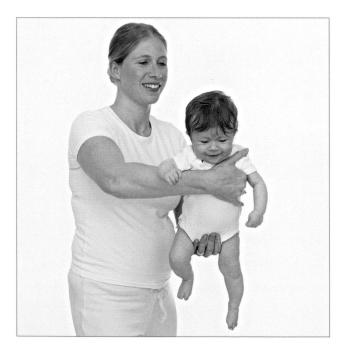

◀ Whooshes from standing

"Whooshes" are an energetic way to calm your baby. Be aware of your baby's mood as she may prefer energetic whooshes or a more gentle movement.

1 From standing, place your strong hand under your baby's seat and your other arm securely across her chest. Your baby should be lying face down.

2 Gently step one leg forward and rhythmically swing your baby back and forward.

3 Repeat the whooshing movement a few times, making sure that as you swing your baby you relax your shoulders and bend your knees to protect your back.

Sitting meditation ▶

Finding a few moments to relax and recharge your batteries sets a good example for your baby and in due course she will learn to relax too in the soothing atmosphere you have created. This takes time, however, so don't give up.

1 Sit in a comfortable position with your baby either on your lap or lying next to you.

2 Exhale deeply two or three times with a few "haaa" breaths, allowing yourself to let go of any tension.

3 Allow your shoulders to drop and soften and make sure you are not holding any tension in your jaw.

4 Allow yourself to relax completely. If you feel you cannot close your eyes, just centre your gaze on a spot in front of you.

5 Take your time to follow your breath, focusing on a few long slow breaths.

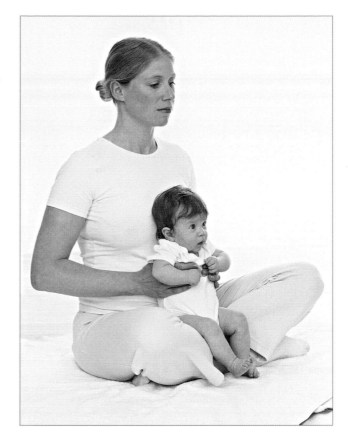

Lying relaxation

If you practise lying relaxation regularly with your baby you will have a chance to bond with her more deeply, free from the worry and clutter of the day. Enjoy a few moments of peace and tranquillity!

1 Lie down on your back with your knees bent. You can have your baby lying against your thighs or lying to the side of you.

2 If you are feeling tense, take a few moments to create tension in your body. As you breathe in, make fists, scrunch up your face, and point your toes. As you breathe out, let go completely and allow your body to soften.

3 If your baby is distressed or fed up, talk softly to her or sing to her. Then hold her gently but firmly.

4 Close and relax your eyes, relax your facial muscles, and check that you are not clenching your teeth. Become aware of your breathing as it is – don't try to change it. Be aware, too, of your baby's breathing. Allow yourself to disengage from the world, letting yourself quieten down, and feel yourself entering deeper into relaxation.

TIP If your baby will not settle, the calming walks with sounds (see page 39) may help to pacify him and release you from tension and worry.

Twinkle, twinkle little star
How I wonder what you are
Up above the world so high
Like a diamond in the sky.

Jane Taylor

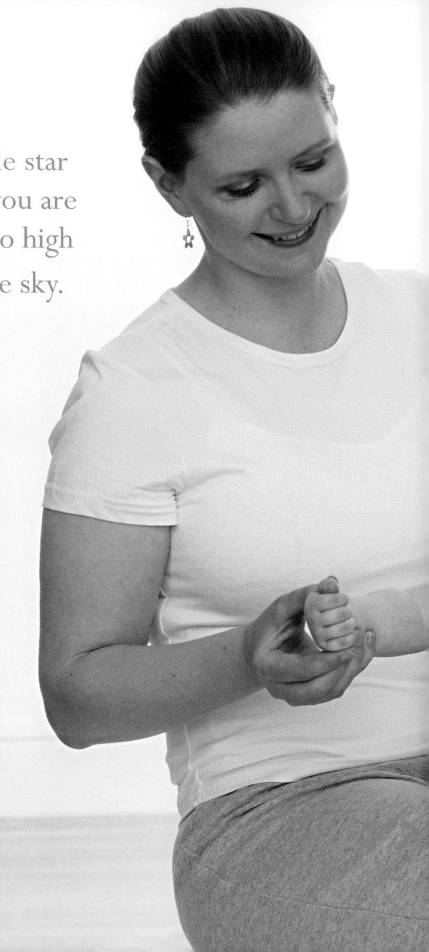

Exercises:
from 6 months to 9 months

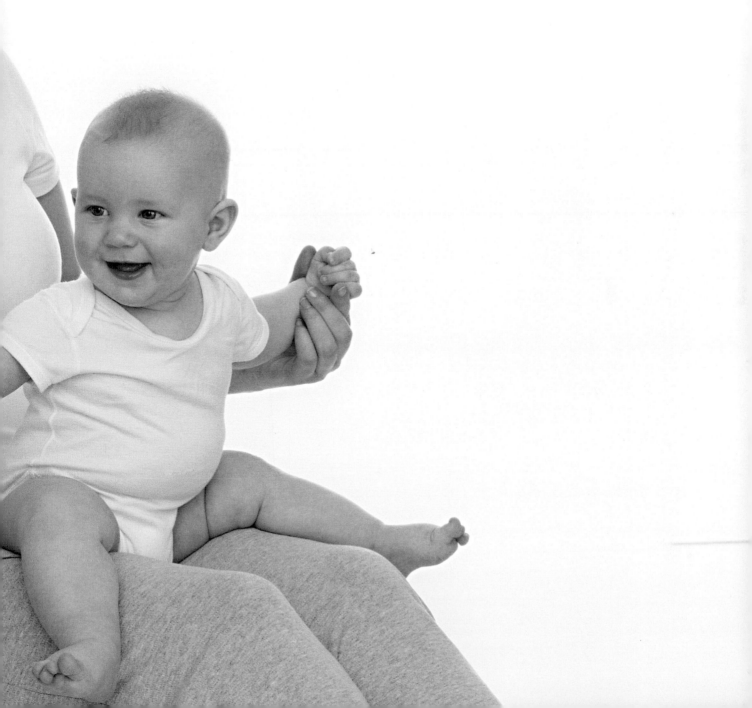

From 6 months to 9 months

Your baby is now bigger and will enjoy more action and activity. You are at the centre of your baby's world and he will love your playful games and songs. He may be sitting up or beginning to crawl. He will be showing you his new talents in each yoga session.

GETTING STARTED – a recap

1 Relax – centre yourself and do a few stretches.

2 Create a setting.

3 Check your position.

4 Make contact.

5 Begin with a warm-up followed by the appropriate sequence for your baby's age and mood.

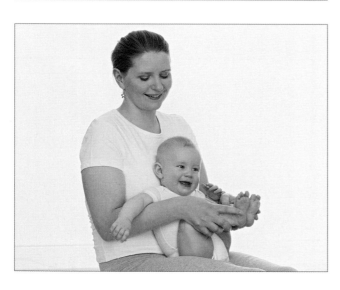

Open and closed legs ▶

1 With your baby still sitting against you, gently hold onto her ankles and open and close his legs.

2 You can make it more fun by saying "*open*" and "*close*" and by gently tapping the soles of his feet together as you close his legs.

Waking-up time

Making contact – see Warm-ups for Babies on page 26.

Gentle dry massage – see Warm-ups for Babies on pages 26–9.

Your baby can sit on your lap for the following exercises and he will enjoy looking around. The more rhythm, songs, and fun you introduce into your sessions, the more reward there will be for him.

◀ Knees to tummy

1 With your baby sitting up against you, gently bring his knees to her tummy.

2 Gently stretch his legs out again and repeat this movement a few times.

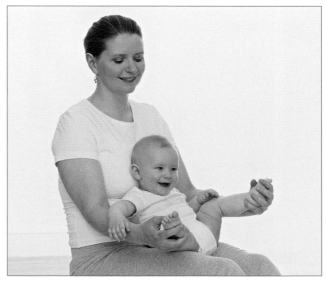

Criss-cross legs ▾

1 Continue the above movements but cross the legs over each other as you bring them together.

2 Make the actions more fun by singing one of your baby's favourite songs to accompany them.

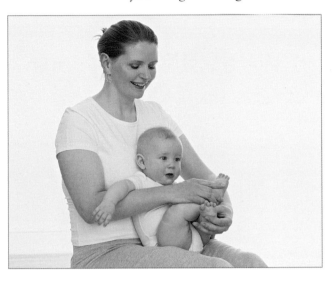

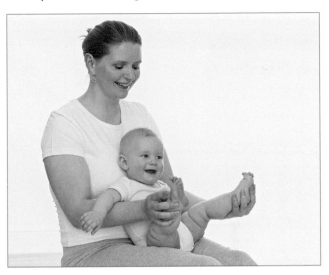

Butterfly and butterfly circles ▸

1 Bring the soles of your baby's feet together.

2 If he is happy, with your hands still holding your baby's feet, gently circle his feet in one direction and then the other.

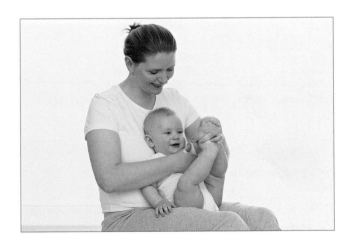

Half lotus

1 With your baby sitting up against you, gently bring one of his feet up toward the opposite inner thigh.

2 Repeat the stretch with the opposite foot.

3 If this exercise comes easily to your baby, and he seems to be enjoying it, you can bring his foot up toward his nose, but be sure never to force this movement. Repeat on the other side.

TIP With all these exercises, never force the movement. As always, try to make any exercise fun but stop at once if your baby doesn't enjoy it.

Arms open and close and "big hug" ▼

1 Holding onto his hands, open your baby's arms wide. You can say "*hello world*" as you do so.

2 Wrap your baby's arms around him very closely while you say "*big hug*".

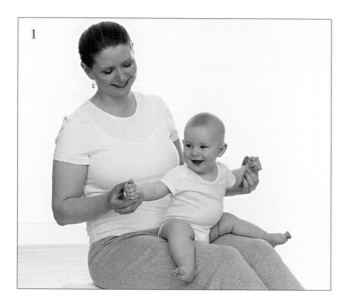

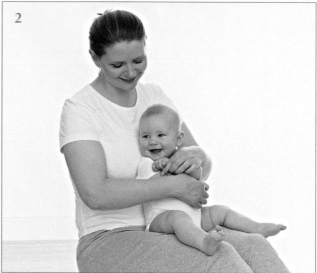

Play time

Your baby will enjoy energetic games and, given the opportunity, will show you all his newly acquired tricks and skills, which may include supported standing and rolling. In the first two of these exercises he will be able to demonstrate his strength and how he can stand on his own two feet.

See-saw balance to standing ▶

1 Sit with your legs out in front of you and with your back as straight as is comfortable. Sit your baby on your lap facing to the side, supporting him with one hand on his chest and the other on his back.

2 Allow your baby to rock forward onto your supporting hand and back onto your other hand. If this feels comfortable, allow him to go all the way forward to standing, steadied by your supporting arm with your other hand resting on his back.

3 Repeat this a few times. Your baby will enjoy being able to work his legs and stand on his own two feet.

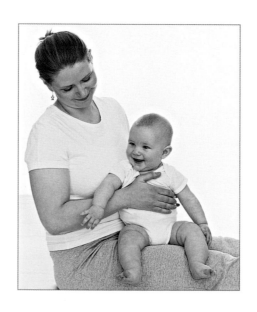

Standing balance ▶

1 Sit in the same position as for the see-saw balance (see opposite page) and place one hand supporting your baby's chest and the other resting on his back.

2 Allow your baby to lift himself up so he is putting all of his weight onto your supporting arm. Keep your other hand gently placed on his back.

3 If your baby is well balanced, you can gently move your hand away from his back.

TIP If you want extra support, place your hand under your baby's bottom

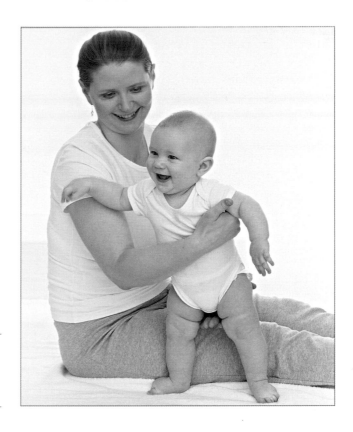

Rolls

See the sequence in play time from 3 months to 6 months on page 49.

Fly baby fly

See the sequence in play time from 3 months to 6 months on page 53.

Warrior with baby

The warrior has both physical and emotional strength. Together in this pose you and your baby will be able to conquer the world!

1 Stand holding your baby however you feel comfortable. Taking your right leg forward, left leg behind, turn the left heel away from you slightly.

2 Turn the upper half of your body so that you are facing forward in the direction of the right foot.

3 Bend the right knee and gently place your baby on your right thigh. Hold onto him with both arms, making sure that he is well supported.

4 If you feel able to do so, keep your strong arm around your baby and extend the other up into the air, stretching into your fingertips. Hold the pose for a moment, breathing long slow breaths. Release your arm down, give your baby a big kiss, and try the pose on the other side.

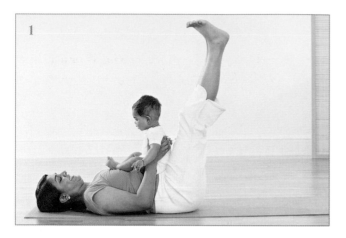

◄ Slow-motion firming with baby

This beautiful and flowing exercise will allow you to strengthen your abdominal muscles. Your baby will love to be included in this sequence. If you suffer from low back pain, avoid this exercise completely.

1 Lie down with your legs bent. Sit your baby on your pelvis with his back against your thighs and support him with your hands. Gently extend both your legs up into the air with your toes toward you and heels away.

2 Keeping both legs straight, maintain your left leg in the air and slowly lower your right leg down to the ground. If you suffer from lower back pain, bend your legs as you bring them down, or avoid this exercise completely.

3 Now lower your left leg so that you are lying completely flat with the small of your back pressed into the ground.

4 Still holding your baby, breathe in and lift yourself up to sitting. Sit up tall with your back straight.

5 Allow your baby to lie on her back against your thighs. Breathe in and as you breathe out lean into a forward bend and give your baby a kiss. Gently lift your baby up to supported sitting and roll yourself down to the ground.

6 Bend your knees and extend both legs up in the air again as in step 1 and repeat the whole sequence, making it as flowing as possible.

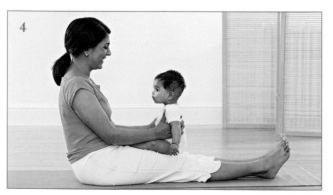

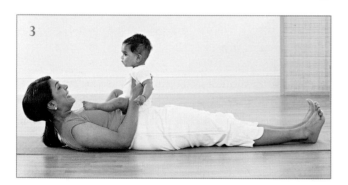

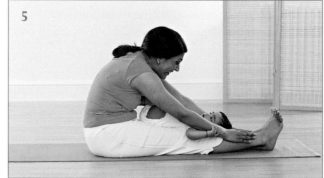

Grizzly time

Sometimes your baby may respond to a little humour when grizzly. Try doing the "sit swings" or a silly dance in the "invigorating walks" to lift an irritable mood. If all else fails, your baby may need some quiet relaxation as in the calming walks or lying relaxation.

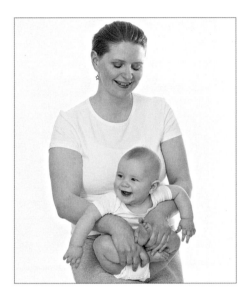

◄ Sit swings

Once your baby can sit securely without support, you can engage him in this game to maintain flexibility in his hip joints. When you are familiar with this exercise you will be able to do it from standing.

1   Sit on your heels with your baby on your lap. Bring your arms under his armpits and hold his ankles. His feet should be together and his knees open.

2   As you pick him up by his ankles, your forearms will work like a safety harness and you can let him lean slightly forward. Now swing him gently from side to side. Repeat this a couple of times.

Invigorating walks

1   Hold your baby at waist level with your forearm across her stomach and your hand tucked under his armpit, or in any relaxed holding position that feels comfortable and secure. Relax your jaw, shoulders, and neck and breathe a few long slow breaths.

2   When you are ready, begin walking and find a comfortable rhythm. This may be a little tap, bending and stretching each leg, or you may prefer a gentle jog or skip. If you are having fun, try a silly dance. As well as experiencing the contrast between stillness and movement, you will both have fun and the movement, free of tension, will energize you.

Calming walks for the older baby

1   Holding your baby at waist level (see above), slowly start to walk.

2   Bring your shoulders to your ears as you breathe in and let them drop as you breathe out. Move your head from side to side, freeing your neck of tension. Your jaw should be loose and your tongue able to move freely in your mouth. Release your breath with a few "haaa" exhalations. Empty your gaze – be aware of you and your baby, together but separate.

3   Pace your walk to your breathing, allowing yourself to be at peace and to disengage from all activity.

Whooshes from standing

See the sequence in Grizzly time: from 3 months to 6 months on page 54.

Lying relaxation

Follow the sequence in Grizzly time: from 3 months to 6 months on page 55.

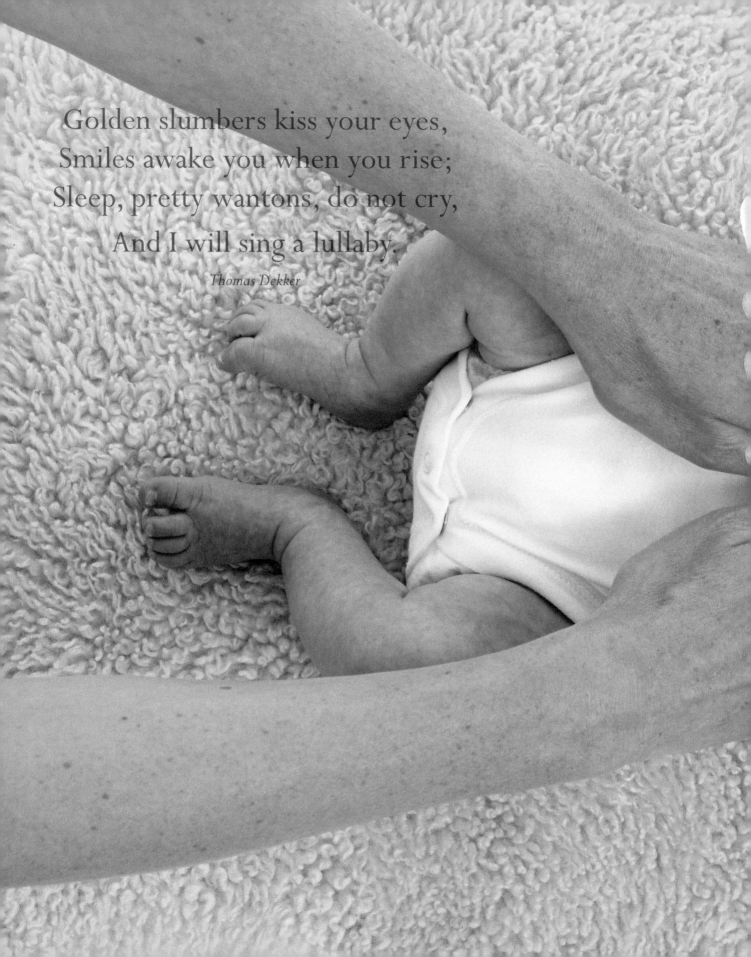

Golden slumbers kiss your eyes,
Smiles awake you when you rise;
Sleep, pretty wantons, do not cry,
And I will sing a lullaby.

Thomas Dekker

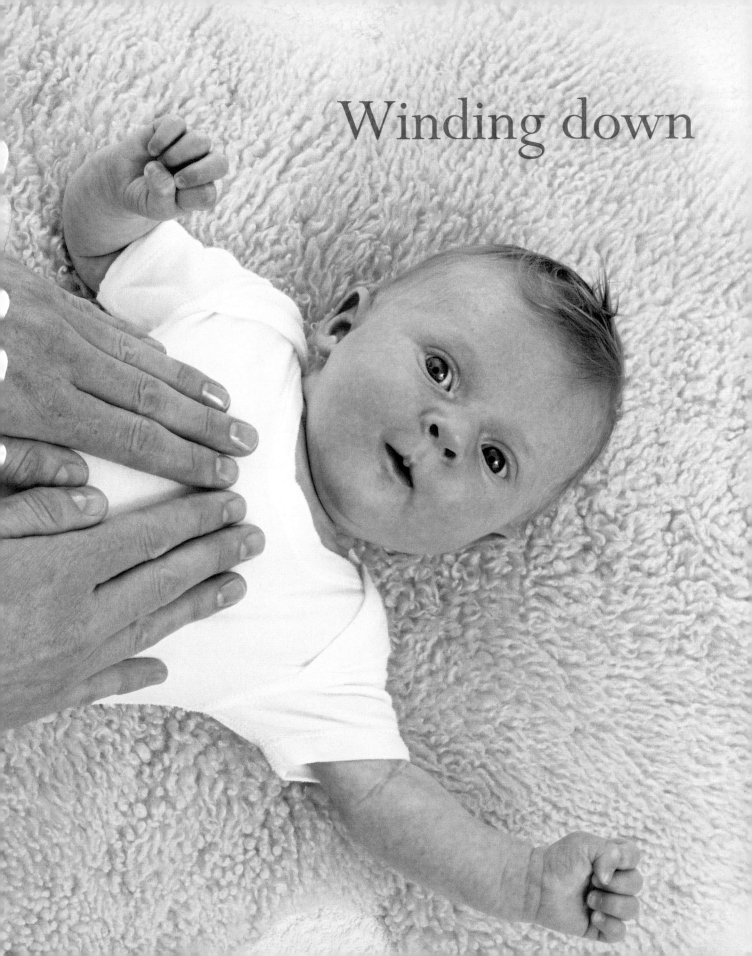

Winding down

The benefits of massage

An effective way to help your baby wind down is to give him a full body massage using an oil. Begin, as in "Warm-ups for babies" (see page 26), by seeking permission, gently asking *"Can I massage you?"*, then giving a long gentle stroke all the way down the body. If your baby seems happy you are ready to begin.

Using massage oils

There are many different oils available, but for massaging your baby choose an organic vegetable-based oil rather than a mineral one. Because they are not readily absorbed into the body, mineral-based oils, which include baby oil, tend to lie on the surface of the skin and block its pores, preventing the skin from breathing. They also inhibit glandular secretions, which keep the skin waterproof and resilient, and thus can be drying. In contrast a pure vegetable, fruit, or nut oil has beneficial properties, such as containing vitamins and minerals that contribute to a healthy skin. Whether you choose grape seed oil, sweet almond oil, or olive oil, it is important to test your baby's skin for reactions by applying the oil to a small patch of skin and leaving it for 24 hours. If your baby reacts, discontinue use immediately.

Legs

INDIAN MILKING

1 Making sure your hands are well oiled, take hold of your baby's leg and shake it gently.

2 Cupping your baby's leg in both hands perform gentle "Indian milking" by sliding one hand down the leg followed by the other. Remember to keep your baby's pelvis on the floor so you don't lift her body with your strokes. Repeat with the other leg.

SQUEEZE AND TWIST

1 Hold your baby's leg in both hands. Turning each hand in the opposite direction in a twisting motion, squeeze your baby's leg slightly as you gently stroke from the thigh to the ankle. Avoid making the twisting movement around your baby's knee joint, and stop if your baby does not like this stroke.

2 Finish the movement by giving a long stroke from the top of the thigh all the way down and allow your baby's leg to drop and relax into your hands. Repeat with the other leg.

ROLLING ▼
Roll each leg between your hands from thigh to ankle.

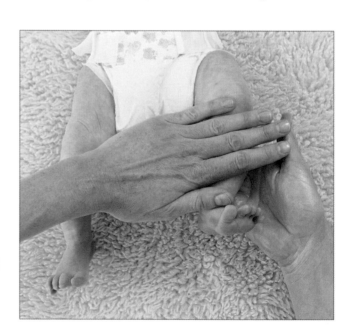

Feet and toes ▶

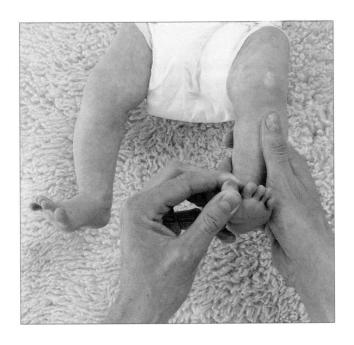

1 With your thumb on the sole of your baby's foot, gently massage each foot from the heel to the toes.

2 Gently squeeze and roll each toe between your index finger and thumb.

3 Gently press the ball of each foot just under the toes.

4 Using your thumbs, one after the other, stroke the top of each foot from the toes toward the ankle.

5 Massage in small circles all around the ankle using your thumbs.

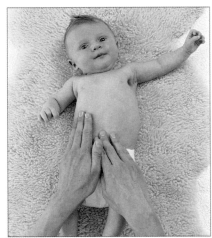

Tummy

This stroke will help to relieve wind and constipation. Place your hands on your baby's tummy, so she knows its time for a tummy massage.

◀ **SUN CIRCLES**
Gently stroke clockwise in a full circle around your baby's navel. Do this lightly several times.

WATER WHEEL
Using the flats of your hands, make paddling strokes on your baby's tummy, one hand following the other, from the chest down.

◀ **THUMBS TO SIDES**
Start with your hands along your baby's sides and your thumbs on her navel. Pull your thumbs out to the sides of her body, making sure you use the flat of the thumbs and do not poke.

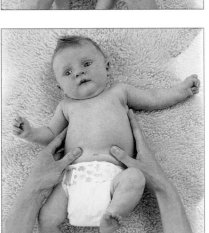

Chest and shoulders

An open chest and shoulders, combined with a relaxed belly, will enable the maximum volume of inspired oxygen to enter the body. Massage of the chest can also help alleviate problems of congestion.

1 Place your relaxed, oiled hands in the centre of your baby's chest.

2 Massage upward and outward over the shoulders, feeling them in the palms of your hands, and back to the centre of the chest. Repeat several times.

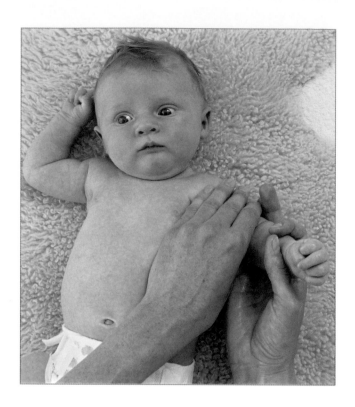

Arms

SQUEEZE AND TWIST ▶
Hold your hands together around your baby's arm, then very gently move your hands in opposite directions, keeping your hands together so as not to twist the elbow joints.

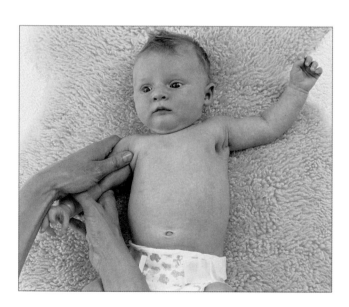

◀ INDIAN MILKING
This helps stress and tension leave the body. Hold your baby's wrist with one hand. Cup the top of her arm with the other and gently pull down toward the wrist. Continue the action, using one hand after the other as though you were milking the arm.

SWEDISH MILKING
This massage uses the same action as "Indian milking" but you start from the wrist and move upward to the shoulder. Stabilize your baby's shoulder with one hand so that you do not pull her body up. Repeat this action several times.

TIP With this stroke you are gently massaging across the muscle, encouraging it to relax.

Hands and fingers ▾

1 Open your baby's hand with your thumbs and roll each finger between your index finger and thumb.

2 Gently massage the whole of her palm using your thumbs. Repeat both steps on the other hand.

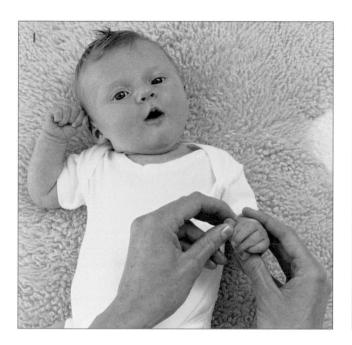

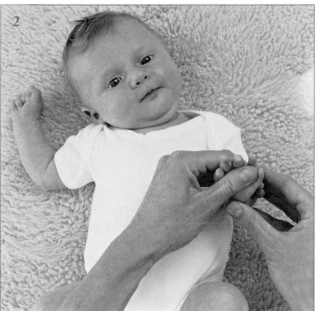

Back

1 Sit with your legs extended and rest your baby on her tummy on your lap.

2 Gently hold your baby's feet with one hand and with the other give her long, slow strokes from the top of her shoulders down her back and legs to her ankles. Repeat several times.

When you have finished massaging your baby, end the "winding down time" with some calming walks, as in "grizzly time" (see page 39 for babies up to 6 months or page 63 for older babies). Don't forget to breathe long slow breaths.

To awaken, sit calmly, letting each breath
clear your mind and open your heart.

The Buddha, translated by Jack Kornfield

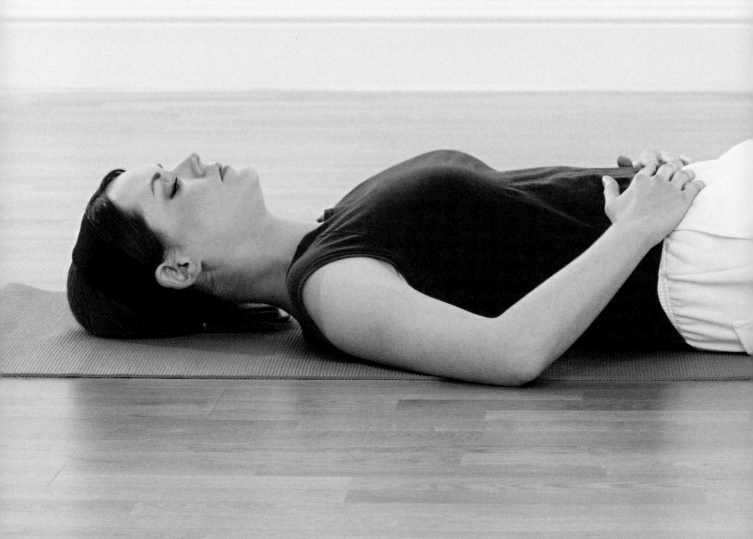

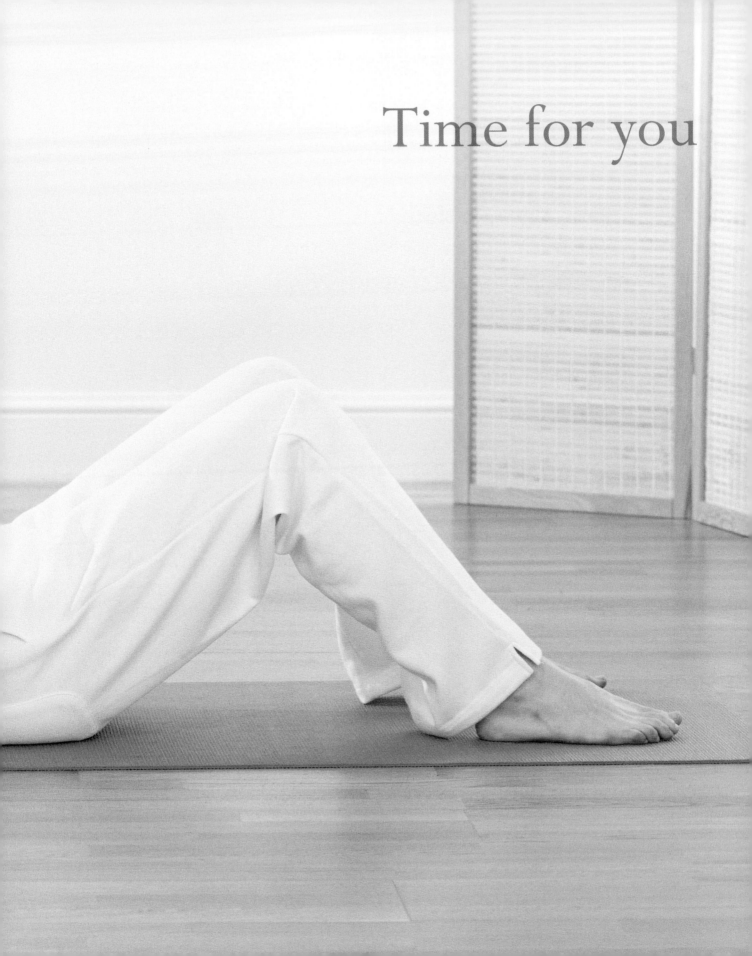

Time for you

From 6 weeks to 3 months

During the 3 months following the birth of your baby your body will be slowly returning to its pre-pregnancy state. The emphasis in these "time for you" exercises is on helping you to gently work on the pelvic floor to regain strength in your abdominal muscles. You will also welcome the breathing exercises and relaxation to help combat the exhaustion you may feel at this time.

Centering and breath awareness ▶

1 Sit in a comfortable upright position. Close your eyes and allow your mind to focus on your breath.

2 Place your hands on your rib cage and gently follow the pattern of your breathing. Be aware of the rising and falling of your rib cage.

3 Be aware of each out breath and focus on completely letting go of any tension.

4 Do not hurry and allow each breath to finish before a new one begins. When you feel ready, slowly open your eyes.

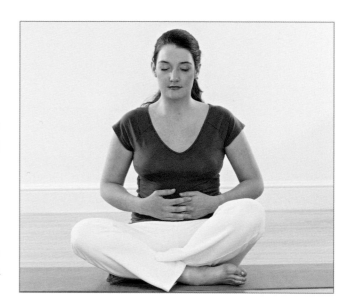

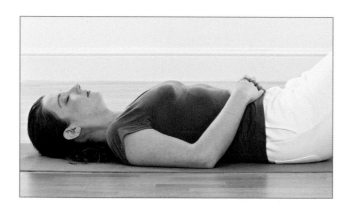

TIP Practise a few rounds of reverse breathing but stop if you feel tired or if you lose your rhythm.

◀ Reverse breathing

You can do this gentle breathing exercise either lying down with your knees bent or sitting upright. It will help tone your deepest abdominal muscles and will also help you to reconnect with your pelvic area. It is especially useful if you have had a Caesarean birth.

1 Begin by being aware of your breath. Focus on the natural flow of your in breath and your out breath.

2 When you are ready, gently deepen your in breath and as you breathe out concentrate on drawing in your tummy to the back of your spine, then release.

3 Repeat this a few times.

Alternate nostril breathing ▶

Alternate nostril breathing acts as a gentle sedative – if you practise it for 5 or 10 minutes it will enable you to turn inward and reach a deep meditative state. It will help you to clarify your thoughts and is especially useful if you are feeling fragmented, nervous, or emotionally upset.

1 Sit in a comfortable upright position.

2 Taking your right hand, place your thumb over your right nostril and your fourth finger over your left nostril. You can rest your second and third fingers on the bridge of your nose.

3 Inhale and exhale. Close the right nostril with your thumb and inhale through your left nostril for a count of five.

4 Close both nostrils, hold for a short moment, then lift your thumb and exhale for a count of five through your right nostril.

5 Inhale through the right nostril for a count of five, hold for a moment, close your right nostril, and exhale through the left nostril for a count of five. This completes one round.

6 Repeat for 4 more rounds.

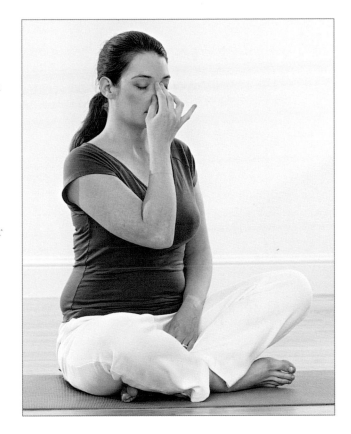

TIP Never force your breathing – it will deepen naturally with practice.

Pelvic floor exercises

A healthy pelvic floor is essential. Try and incorporate this pose into your daily life, taking any opportunity you can to do this exercise.

1 Choose a comfortable position. You may prefer to be lying down or in a semi-squat position with your knees slightly bent, but you can actually practise this exercise anywhere.

2 Begin by focusing on your pelvic floor muscles and your breathing. Toward the end of each exhalation contract your pelvic floor muscles, drawing them firmly toward the uterus. Hold tight and then release gently as you inhale.

3 Repeat up to 20 times, working your pelvic floor muscles with the rhythm of your breathing.

Lying spinal twist ▼

This is a centering pose that will calm your mind.

1 Lie on your back on the floor with your knees bent, feet together, and arms out to the sides. Keep the back of your waist flat on the floor.

2 Breathe deeply into the abdomen. As you exhale, allow your knees to drop down toward the floor on the right-hand side, keeping them together as you slowly lower them down. Then turn your head to the left, breathing evenly.

3 As you inhale, gently bring your knees and head back to the centre while keeping the rest of your body stable.

4 Repeat the exercise, this time moving your legs to the left and your head to the right. Repeat several times on each side.

5 Finish by hugging your knees to your chest and gently rocking from side to side, which will release your back.

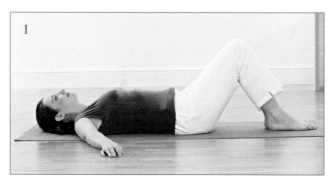

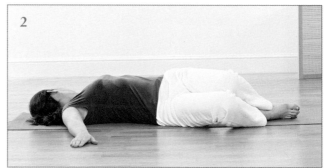

Swan stretch ▼

This pose will stretch your spine and help to remove any stiffness in your shoulder girdle. Try and lengthen your spine and relax your shoulders as you exhale.

1 Sit on your heels as straight as you can. Lengthen through the spine and look straight ahead.

2 As you breathe in, stretch your arms up above your head.

3 As you exhale, lower your arms forward and raise your hips so that you come up onto your hands and knees. Your hands should be shoulder-width apart and your knees under your hips.

4 On your next exhalation, sit back on your heels. Feel the stretch through your shoulders and back.

5 Creep your hands forward to increase the stretch and take several long slow breaths.

6 Slowly return to the starting position when you are ready and repeat the exercise in your own time.

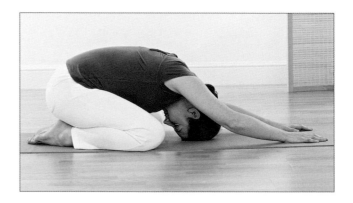

Cat pose ▼

Enjoy the gentle stretching of your spine in this pose. Remember to focus on your breath.

1 Start on all fours with your knees under your hips. Keep the shoulders, elbows, and wrists in line and spread your fingers. Lengthen through your arms as you bring your shoulders away from your ears. Your back should be relaxed and run in a straight line from your hips to the back of your head.

2 Breathing in deeply, slowly tilt the tail bone upward and extend the chest down between the arms, making the spine concave, as you lift your head to look directly ahead. Pause briefly.

3 Exhale slowly, tucking the tail bone under and drawing the abdomen back to round the lower back as you gradually arch through the spine and lower your head.

4 On your next in breath, slowly tilt the tail bone as in step 2. Repeat the whole exercise a couple of times and then rest forward in the "swan stretch" (see opposite).

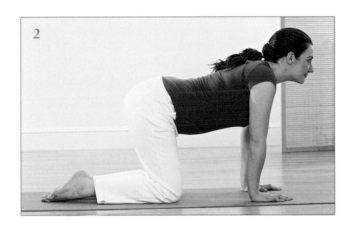

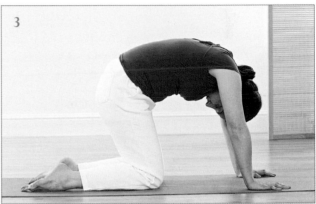

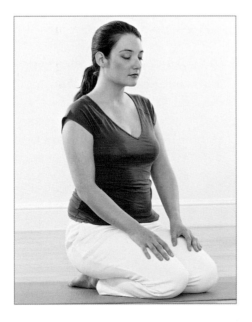

◄ Humming breath

Humming breath can promote a relaxing inner peace and is a good antidote to stress, anger, and anxiety.

1 Sit in a comfortable position with a straight spine. Place a cushion under you if you need to.

2 Close your eyes and be aware of your breath. When you are ready, breathe in deeply. As you breathe out, keep the mouth closed, jaw relaxed, and teeth slightly apart, and make a deep, soft humming sound.

3 Allow the sound to fade at the end of the exhalation and breathe normally. Repeat 5 times. When you are finished, allow your breath to return to normal.

From 3 months to 6 months

You may be feeling more energized and less tired than you did during the first 3 months. Now is the time to introduce slightly bigger stretches, especially standing poses, as you regain your strength.

Tadasana – the mountain pose

This is the basis of the classical yoga poses, focusing on balance, posture, physical alignment, inner strength, and confidence.

1   Stand up straight with your feet parallel, hip width apart, and your ears, tops of shoulders, hips, and ankles in alignment. Press your feet into the ground and lift upward through your body.

2   You should feel balanced in all directions and your head should feel as if it is suspended by a thread from the ceiling. Look straight ahead, relax, and breathe easily.

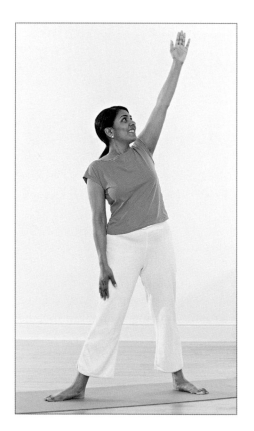

Archer pose

This pose will strengthen your leg muscles and open your shoulder joints and chest.

1   Stand in "Tadasana" then place your feet about 1m (3ft) apart. Turn your right foot out and left foot in.

2   Inhale and raise your arms open to shoulder level. Exhale, bend your right knee, and turn your head right, extending both arms as far as you can.

3   Inhale, straighten your legs, centre your head, and turn the left foot out, right foot in. Exhale and stretch to the left. Continue, alternating sides.

◄ Gentle triangle

This ancient pose, which replicates the innate stability of a triangle, will improve the flexibility of your torso, open your hip area, and strengthen your arms, legs, ankles, and feet. Only stretch as far as you can go – never force the movement.

1   Begin in "Tadasana", as above. With your feet apart and arms extended, tilt your body to the right.

2   Breathe naturally and allow your right hand to slide down your right leg to the point where you feel you cannot go any further down without leaning forward.

3   Keeping your weight on your left leg, inhale, and stretch into the fingertips of your left hand. Look at the left hand and stretch further as you exhale.

4   Come back to centre and repeat on the left side.

Relaxed forward bend ▶

After doing the standing poses opposite, you can relax your body forward.

1 Stand in "Tadasana" (see opposite) then gently lower your arms to the floorand flop into a forward bend. Relax your neck.

2 Swing your head and shoulders gently from side to side to ease and release your lower neck.

3 Bend your knees as you breathe in to come back up.

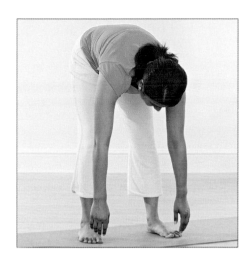

◀ **Leg stretch**

This is a beautiful stretch that you can practise anywhere that you have a flat surface of the right height – the kitchen table, sofa, or a chair, perhaps.

1 Carefully place one leg on a table or a chair, making sure the surface isn't too high. Both legs should be straight. Flex the toes of the raised foot toward you.

2 As you inhale, raise both arms above your head. Exhale and stretch further. When you are ready, lower your arms on the out breath and slide one hand down your leg, keeping your back straight.

3 With each out breath, try and extend a bit further. Keep your head relaxed. When you are ready, change legs and repeat.

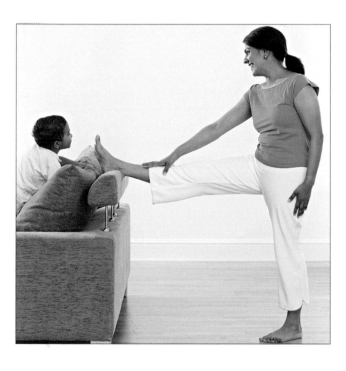

Eagle pose

This is a slightly more advanced pose for those who have practised yoga before. This pose focuses on "closing" the body after you have had your baby.

1 Stand in "Tadasana" (see opposite) and focus on your breathing. Rest your hands on top of your hips and breathe in. As you breathe out, bend your knees and wrap your right leg around your left leg, tucking your right foot behind your left calf.

2 When you feel ready, raise your bent left arm in front of your face and bring your bent right arm around it. Bring your palms together.

3 Sit down as if on an invisible chair and focus on your fingers directly in front of your face.

4 When you feel ready, repeat on the other side.

Back stretch ▶

This is perfect to stretch and lengthen your spine. Most mothers enjoy this pose, especially if they spend a lot of time carrying their baby. This stretch is also done against a table or counter.

1 Put your hands on the table, bend at the hips, and walk backward until you can stretch your spine out horizontally. Try to avoid tensing your head, jaw, and shoulders.

2 To enjoy a bigger stretch, bend your knees and push your bottom out to pull the base of the spine further away from your shoulders. Breathe long slow breaths and hold the stretch for as long as is comfortable.

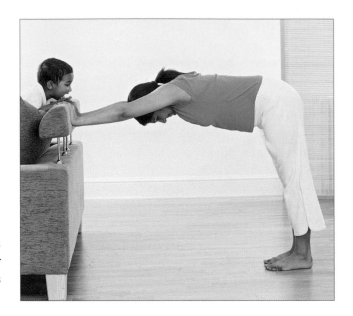

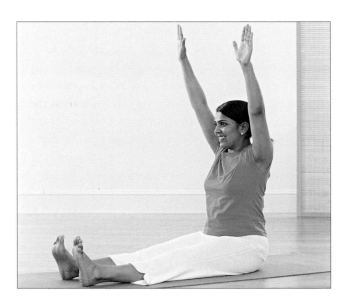

Rolling cat

Focus on deep long slow breathing and release any tension or anxiety as you exhale.

1 Start on all fours, as in the "cat pose" (see page 75).

2 Round your back, tucking your chin in, as you breathe out.

◀ Dandasana with raised arms

This is a traditional yoga position that will stretch the back of your legs and your spine.

1 Sit on a mat with your legs stretched out and your toes pointing to the ceiling. Place your hands near your bottom and use them to push your spine upright. Focus on your breathing.

2 Bring the palms of your hands into a prayer pose (see page 22). On your next in breath, stretch your arms up above your head. Breathing out, lower your arms down. Repeat a couple of times.

3 Bring your bottom to your heels and roll your nose across the ground as you breathe in.

4 Round your back again, tucking your chin in as you breathe out.

5 Finally, sit back on your heels with your forehead on the floor and your arms beside you, palms facing up.

Cat balance ▶

This balance will help develop stability in your hip and shoulder joints while stretching your body diagonally.

1 Start on all fours with your knees under your hips. Your shoulders, elbows, and wrists should be in line and your back relaxed and in a straight line from your hips to the back of your head. Breathe easily.

2 Draw your tummy in and raise your right arm and left leg simultaneously as you breathe in. Pause briefly, then lower them as you breathe out.

3 Repeat with the left arm and right leg, then several times on each side.

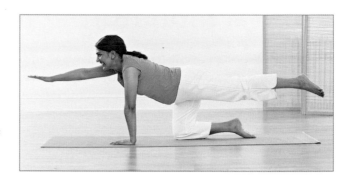

TIP Finish this stretch by resting in the "child's pose" (see page 24). Breathe deeply and relax in this position for a few moments.

Lying relaxation ▼

Relaxing at the end of a yoga session will give your body and mind a chance to absorb the benefits of your practice – once learned, these relaxation techniques can be used anywhere and anytime to help you "let go".

1 Lie straight and flat on a mat with your feet hip width apart and your arms away from your body. Stretch through your arms to your fingertips then let your arms and shoulders relax. Stretch out your legs and flex your toes toward you, then let go. Be aware of your surroundings then close your eyes.

2 Be aware of the back of your head and let it sink down. Let your eyes feel heavy beneath the eyelids. Relax your jaw so that your teeth part slightly and smile a little to relax your face. Swallow and let your neck relax. Relax your right hand, arm, shoulder, and the right side of your trunk. Relax your right hip, buttock, leg, and foot. Then do the same on the left side of your body. Feel that your body is now relaxed from your head to your feet.

3 Feel your chest and abdomen rise as you breathe in then sink down as you breathe out. Be aware of new energy as you inhale and of letting go as you exhale.

4 When you are ready, become aware again of your surroundings. Wiggle your fingers and toes. Take a couple of deep breaths, then stretch and yawn or sigh. Turn onto your side then slowly sit up.

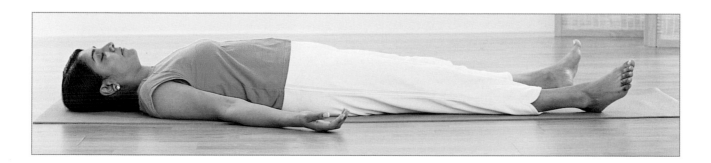

From 6 months to 9 months

You may be feeling completely restored to your former self or slowly beginning to feel that way and your yoga practice can now focus on strengthening your muscles and improving your alignment. With practice you will feel increasingly capable, but don't forget that relaxation is still just as important.

Centering and breath awareness ▶

1 Lie in a comfortable upright position. Slowly allow your mind to focus on your breathing.

2 Place your hands on your rib cage and gently follow the pattern of your breath. Be aware of the rising and falling of your rib cage.

3 Be aware of each out breath, allowing you to completely let go of tension.

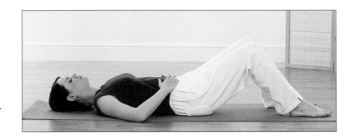

4 Do not hurry – allow each breath to finish before a new one begins. When you feel ready, slowly open your eyes.

Standing forward bend ▼

This is an inverted pose – one in which your head is lower than your heart. It is a relaxing pose that will increase circulation and can relieve fatigue. It will also lengthen and align your spine, reduce lower back pain, and stretch the backs of your legs and your hamstring muscles.

1 Stand in "Tadasana" (see page 76) with your feet slightly apart. Take your hands to the crease at the tops of your legs where they join your torso.

2 Lift your breast bone up and away from the floor to lengthen the front of your body. As you breathe out, fold forward from the hips, bending your knees slightly.

3 With your knees still bent, allow your spine to relax and lengthen as gravity pulls your head and upper body down toward the floor. Let your upper body hang from your hips, press your feet into the floor, and lift your tail bone upward so that you lengthen through the backs of your legs.

4 Bring your arms above your head and hold onto your elbows. Stay here for several breaths.

5 When you are ready, bend your knees, put your hands on your hips, and slowly come back up to a standing position.

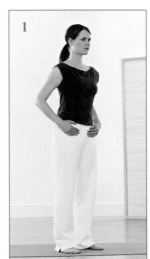
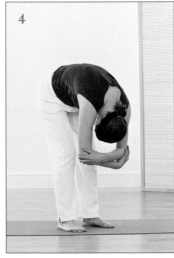

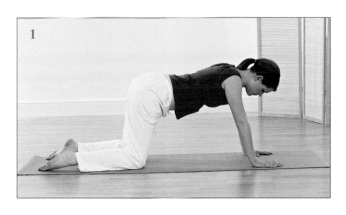

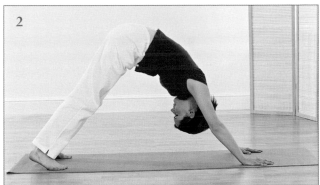

Downward-facing dog ▲

This energizing pose will release tension in your shoulders, strengthen your arms and legs, lengthen your hamstrings and Achilles tendons, and increase flexibility in your ankles. With practice you will be able to bring your heels to the floor. Do not attempt this pose if you suffer from glaucoma.

1 Start on all fours and spread out your fingers and tuck your toes under.

2 Breathe in as you straighten your legs and lift your bottom up toward the ceiling. (You can bend your knees if you need to.) Breathe out as you lower your heels to the ground. Draw your head between your arms and look toward your navel.

3 Hold the pose as long as you feel comfortable. When you have finished, come back to all fours then rest in the child's pose (see page 24).

Triangle pose (Trikonasana) ▶

This is the same as the gentle triangle (see page 76) but a little more demanding. This pose builds physical strength, improves mood, and promotes balance.

1 Standing with your feet about 1m (3ft) apart, bring your arms together in front of your chest.

2 As you breathe in, lift your arms to shoulder height. Turn your right foot out and your left foot in. As you exhale, extend your right arm out as far as it will go. Bend your left arm and rest the palm of your hand on the small of your back.

3 Breathe out and lower your right arm down your leg. Breathe in and extend your left arm straight above your head. Turn your head to look up at your hand.

4 To come out of the pose, breathe in and return to an upright position, with your arms outstretched

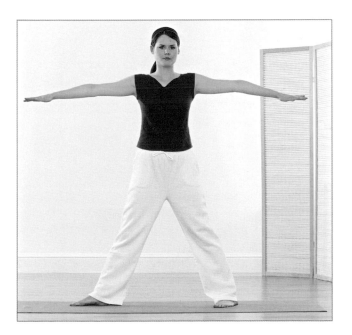

and your feet facing forward. Bring your palms back together to your chest. Take a long slow breath and, when you are ready, repeat on the other side.

Upward-facing dog ▶

This pose gives a powerful upward lift through the front of the body, extending the spine and opening the chest to encourage rib-cage breathing.

1 Start on your hands and knees with your arms shoulder width apart and your feet and knees a little apart. Spread your fingers.

2 Tuck your toes under, breathe in deeply and as you breathe out allow your hips to sink forward and down. Keep your arms straight, the insides of your elbows facing each other, and look straight ahead. Roll your shoulders back and down. Bring your lower legs off the floor if you are able to. If this is too strenuous bring your knees to the ground. Look forward and breathe steadily.

3 To come out of the pose, bend the arms to lower yourself to the floor. Lie on your front, arms beside your body, palms facing up, resting with your head turned to the side.

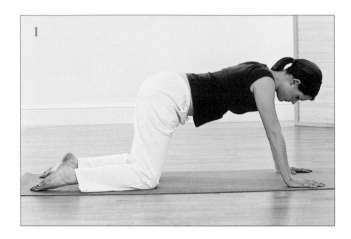

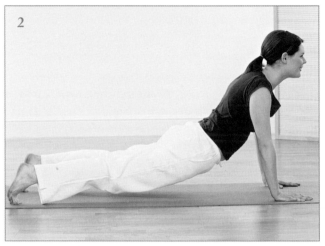

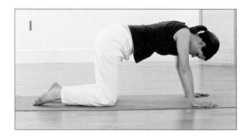

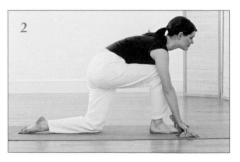

◀ Lunge warrior

This pose will provide a powerful stretch through the thigh and hip, extend your spine, and open your chest.

1 Begin on all fours with your palms pressed to the floor and fingers spread.

2 As you exhale, take your right leg forward between your hands, so that your knee is directly above your heel. Balance yourself with your fingertips if you need to.

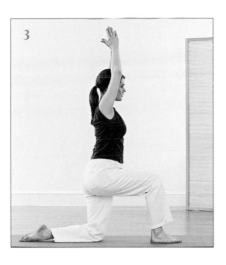

3 With your next in breath, straigthen your body upright and carefully raise your arms above your head with palms touching. Breathe a couple of long slow breaths.

4 Repeat on the other side then rest forward in the child's pose (see page 24).

Cobra ▾

The cobra will extend your spine, strengthening the muscles in your back and stretching the front of your body. It will also open your chest and release tension in your shoulders.

1 Lie on your front on a yoga mat with your forehead on the floor and your feet hip width apart. Let your arms rest straight by your sides, with the palms of your hands facing upward, and stretch your feet along the floor.

2 Place your hands under your shoulders, spread your fingers, keep the elbows close to the body, and roll your shoulders back. Tuck your tail bone under.

3 As you breathe in, slide your forehead forward to lift your forehead, nose, chin, shoulders, and chest. Use your back muscles to lift your upper body off the floor. There should be no feeling of strain and you should breathe easily.

4 Repeat the pose once or twice, resting in between with your forehead on the floor and your arms beside you.

5 When you are finished, rest in the starting position but with your head turned to the side.

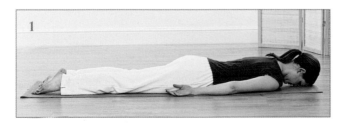

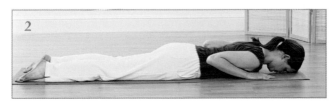

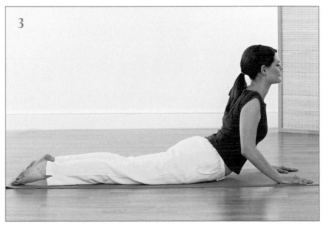

Slow motion firming ▼

This is a particularly valuable exercise as it tones and stretches the whole body. It should be performed as one continuous slow flowing motion.

TIP If this exercise feels too strenuous, omit it from your practice until you feel stronger. Avoid it if you suffer from lower back pain.

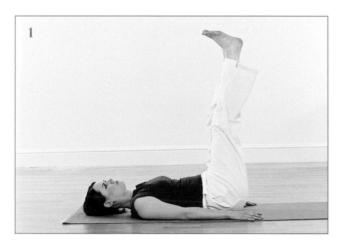

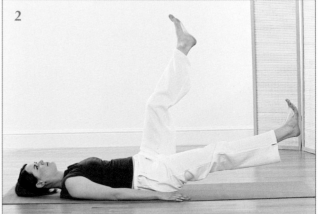

1 Lie on your back on a mat with your feet together. Your arms should be beside you and the palms of your hands toward the floor. Bend your knees in toward your chest then extend them into the air.

2 Slowly lower your right leg down to the ground and, as soon as it touches the floor, begin to slowly lower your left leg so that both your legs are lying straight on the floor.

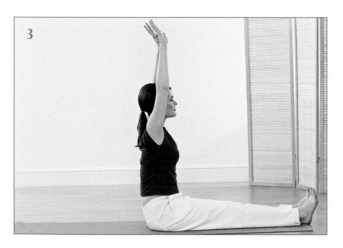

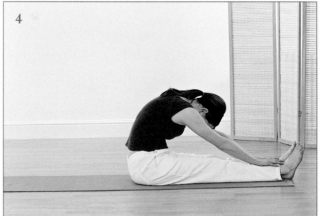

3 Reach forward with your arms and try to sit up without using your hands to help you. Raise your arms straight up above your head and straighten your back.

4 Bring your arms down, reach forward, and firmly take hold of your legs as close to your ankles as you can comfortably manage. Gently let your head relax forward in a forward bend.

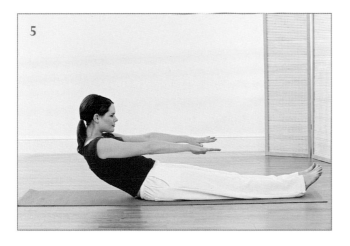

5

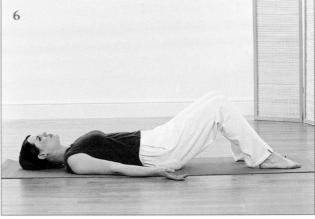

6

5 Roll slowly back down your spine, one vertebra at a time. Keep your arms straight out in front of you, above your thighs, to ensure that your shoulders stay rounded, and push away with your feet to control the movement. Roll back slowly all the way to the floor.

6 When your head touches the ground, place your arms down beside you, with the palms of your hands facing upward, and bend your knees ready to repeat the entire movement.

Lying abdominal breathing ▶

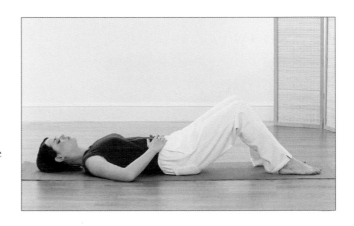

This practice will relax your body and mind and help you to let go of any tension.

1 Lie on your back with your knees bent and your feet about hip width apart. Allow your breath to settle into a smooth, natural rhythm. Become aware of the rise and fall of your abdomen as you breathe in and out. Focus on your out breath and gradually allow it to become longer than your in breath.

2 Try and make your out breath longer and slower by imagining you are drawing your abdomen toward the base of your spine as you exhale. Relax as you breathe in, allowing the abdomen to swell out. After a while, relax and allow your breathing to return to normal.

Routines for you

Here are three examples of mini yoga sequences. If you wish you can invent your own, beginning with centering, followed by two or three asanas (poses or movements) from the correct section, and finishing with a breathing or relaxation session. Each session should leave you feeling balanced and relaxed.

From 6 weeks to 3 months
(5 to 10 minute mini yoga session)

- Centering and breath awareness (see page 72)
- Reverse breathing (see page 72)
- Prayer pose stretch (see page 22)
- Cat pose (see page 75)
- Swan stretch (see page 74)
- Alternate nostril breathing (see page 73)

From 3 months to 6 months
(5 to 10 minute mini yoga session)

- Centering and breath awareness (see page 72)
- Gentle triangle (see page 76)
- Relaxed forward bend (see page 77)
- Leg stretch (see page 77)
- Back stretch (see page 78)
- Lying relaxation (see page 79)

From 6 months to 9 months
(10 to 15 minute mini yoga session)

- Centering and breath awareness (see page 80)
- Modified sun salutations (see page 87)
- When you feel strong, move to sun salutations (see page 88). Begin with one round and build up to three to four rounds.
- End with lying relaxation (see page 79)

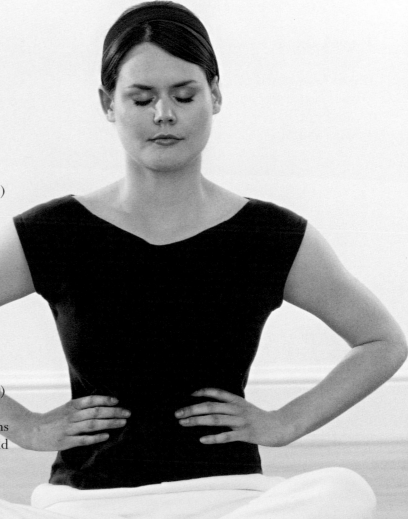

Modified sun salutations ►

This routine is ideal if you find the full sun salutations (see pages 88–9) too demanding. It will help you gain the strength and flexibility required for the full sequence and is great for energizing your body.

1 Stand in "Tadasana" (see page 76), placing your hands in front of you in the prayer pose.

2 Inhale and lift your arms above your head with your palms facing each other but not touching.

3 Exhale and fold forward at the waist into the forward bend, tucking your chin under and bending your knees slightly. If you can touch the floor, try to rest your palms on either side of your feet.

4 Inhale and straighten your legs. Engage your abdominal muscles and slowly raise your upper body to an upright position. Exhale.

5 Inhale and lift your hands over your head with your palms facing but not touching, as in step 2. Bend your upper torso back slightly.

6 Exhale and lower your upper body, bending at the waist as in step 3. Inhale, engage your abdominal muscles, and lift your chin. Keeping your knees soft, return your body to an upright position. Raise your arms, with palms facing but not touching.

7 Exhale and return to the start position with your hands in front of your chest in the prayer pose. Repeat the whole sequence a couple of times.

TIP If you cannot manage to reach the floor in the forward bend, you can bend your knees a bit more. With practice your flexibility will improve.

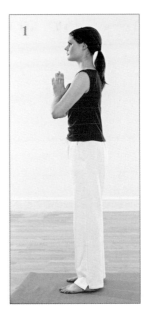

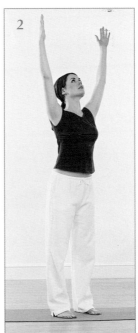

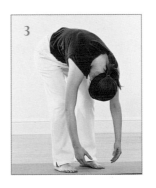

Sun salutations

This sequence will energize and stretch your whole body. Go at your own speed and after completing the sequence on the right side, repeat it on the other. If it feels too difficult, try the modified sun salutation (see page 87) and gradually build up to the full sequence.

TIP These "sun salutations" include many of the poses and movements shown in this chapter. It is a good idea to familiarize yourself with these before attempting to combine them here.

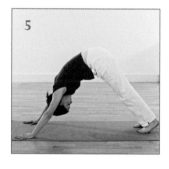

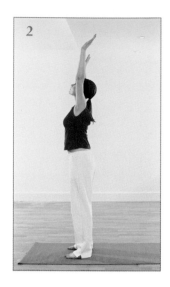

1   Stand up straight with your feet about hip width apart and your palms in the prayer pose in front of your chest. Focus on your breathing.

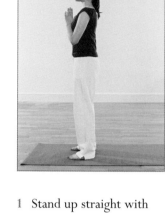

2   As you breath in, take your arms out to the sides of your body, turning the palms out, then lift both arms above your head. Open your chest as you look up at your hands.

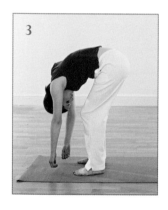

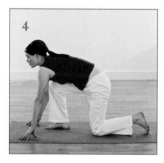

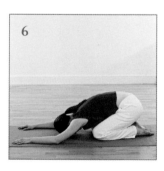

3   Breathing out, fold forward from the hips into a relaxed forward bend (see page 77). Bend your knees if you need to. Hold this pose for a couple of breaths.

4   As you exhale, come into the "lunge warrior" pose (see page 82). Take a large step back with your right foot, lower your right knee to the floor, and rest your chest on your left thigh. Look straight ahead and breathe a couple of long slow breaths.

5   On an out breath, step your left foot back to come into a "downward-facing dog" (see page 81). Ease your heels to the ground but do not force them. Relax your head and hold this pose for a couple of breaths.

6   Bring your knees to the floor, keeping your hands still, as you breathe out. Rest in this "swan stretch" (see page 74) for a few breaths.

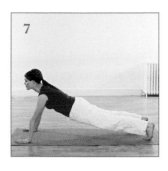

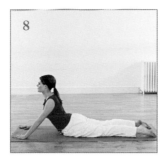

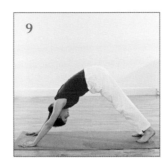

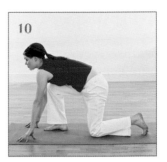

7 Breathe in, bring your body forward, and lift your legs and torso off the floor, tucking your toes under, in the "upward-facing dog" (see page 82). If you are finding this difficult, you can bring your knees to the ground, which will be less strenuous.

8 Breathing in, lower yourself into the "cobra" pose (see page 83) and take a couple of long slow breaths.

9 Breathing out, tuck your toes under and move into the "downward-facing dog" again. Hold this pose for 2 or 3 breaths.

10 Inhale as you step your right foot between your hands to come back into the "lunge warrior". Hold the pose while you breathe a couple of long slow breaths.

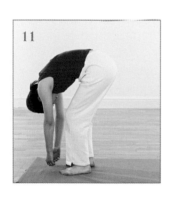

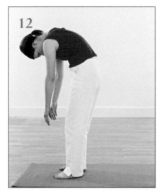

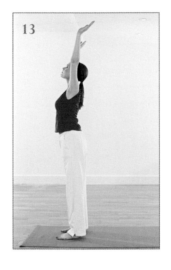

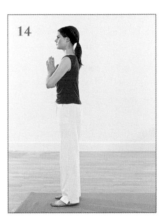

11 As you exhale, bring your right foot forward to join your left foot and come into a forward bend, bending your knees if you need to. Relax your neck and take a couple of breaths.

12 Roll your body up slowly as you breathe in, keeping your knees bent, until you are completely upright.

13 Breathe in, take your arms out to the side of your body, and lift both arms up above your head. Look up.

14 As you breathe out, bring your arms down in front of your chest in the prayer pose. Breathe normally for a few minutes then, when you are ready, repeat on the other side.

Glossary

Abdominal breathing   A breathing technique in which the chest remains largely still and the abdominal muscles do the work. The belly is pushed out to breathe in, and drawn in to breathe out, which lowers and raises the diaphragm. The technique strengthens the abdominal muscles.

Achilles tendon   A popular term used to describe the large tendon running from the back of the calf to the heel bone. It is named after the Greek hero Achilles, who was said to be vulnerable only in his heel.

Alternate nostril breathing   A breathing exercise, in yoga also called "Nadi Shodhana", that is used to induce relaxation and improve mental function. One nostril is closed and the breath is inhaled through the other one. This nostril is then closed and the breath is exhaled through the first one. The process is then repeated.

Asana   A body pose or posture used in yoga. It forms a suffix in the names of various yoga poses, for example Tadasana (the mountain pose) and Shavasana.

Ashtanga yoga   A strong type of yoga (not used in mother and baby yoga) that involves intense aerobic movements. It is sometimes also called power yoga.

Basic yoga breathing   Yoga breathing begins with a slow calm exhalation of breath, which relaxes the inspiratory muscles. This empties the lungs in readiness for proper breathing. The yogic breath involves chest, diaphragm, and abdomen working in unison. The ribs are expanded without straining and the lungs allowed to fill completely by raising the collar bones. The diaphragm is then slowly lowered, allowing air to enter the lungs. As breath is inhaled, the abdomen also expands. The whole process should be silent, single, and rhythmical.

Bhagavad Gita   A key ancient Hindu scripture. The name meas the "lord's song". It contains teachings on yoga, a word that means "union".

Bikram yoga   A type of vigorous yoga (not used in mother and baby yoga) that is practised in a hot room and involves a lot of sweating.

Caesarean birth   A planned or emergency surgical procedure that can be used when a vaginal birth is not advised. A cut about 20cm (8in) long is made in the lower abdomen and the womb is opened to release the baby.

Colic   Babies with colic suffer bouts of uncontrollable crying that can last for several hours and occur several times a week. Colic usually occurs in babies from about 3 weeks to 3 months old and has several possible causes, including stress associated with life outside the womb and, less commonly, allergies or bowel troubles.

Dandasana   A standard yoga pose, or asana, this is the foundation seated pose, often called the "staff pose". It is performed sitting upright on a firm surface with the legs extended out in front and pressed into the floor and toes pointing up. The back should be straight and the body weight on the front of the sitting bones. The hands should be palm down on the floor beside the hips.

Glaucoma   A type of eye disease affecting the optic nerve that can damage vision. In the most common form of the disease, the eyes' drainage channels become blocked over time, raising the pressure inside the eyeball.

Hamstrings   A popular term used to describe the muscles at the back of the thigh. These muscles include the *biceps femoris, semitendinosus,* and *semimembranosus.*

Hatha yoga   A popular type of yoga that uses breathing practices, or "pranayama", and a wide range of body postures. Ha-tha means "sun"-"moon" – a fusion of opposites.

Indian milking   A gentle rhythmic massage technique using both hands that imitates the action you might make in milking a cow.

Limbic system   A part of the brain that is involved with basic urges and feelings, such as hunger, thirst, emotion, and recognition of facial gestures such as smiles.

Mula bandha   A yoga technique that involves a gentle lifting of the pelvic floor combined with reverse breathing. In classical yoga a "bandha" is a lock or valve that channels or releases body energy.

Namaste A gesture made by bringing together the palms of both hands before the heart with fingers pointing up and head slightly bowed. Derived from the Sanskrit words "nama" meaning "bend" and "te" meaning "you", it is used as a humble and straightforward greeting.

Om A chant consisting of three sounds, "a", "u", and "m", om is a sacred sound in ancient Indian religion that is said to drive away cluttered thoughts, bring relaxation, and renew energy. The om represents the everything from which the universe was made.

Pelvic floor A group of muscles in the base of the pelvis, important in childbirth, sexual function, urination, and defecation. The sling of muscles stretches from the pubic bone to the tail bone, supports the pelvic contents, and has openings for the bladder, bowel, and womb.

Postnatal depression Unlike the "baby blues", which are mild and very common in the few days after giving birth, postnatal depression is longer-lasting, deeper, and may need professional treatment. In the "baby blues" many women experience mood swings, crying, irritability, restlessness, and lowness. In postnatal depression there may be stronger feelings of anxiety, despair, anger, and sadness that can last for months. There may also be changes in weight, inability to concentrate, feelings of worthlessness, and a loss of interest in normal daily life.

Prana An ancient Hindu term denoting life force energy that is found in all aspects of nature. It is the vital air or breath of the human body and the life force of the universe.

Pranayama Breathing techniques used in yoga to calm the mind and strengthen the prana (life energy).

Prefrontal cortex Part of the frontal lobe of the brain, often regarded as the "higher brain". It is involved with emotional responses, memory, and controlling complex body movements.

Reverse breathing A breathing practice that helps to restore deep muscle tone and that is especially helpful after Caesarean birth. Breath is inhaled in the normal way and as it is exhaled the navel is drawn toward the spine.

Rib cage breathing A breathing technique in which all the muscles of the chest wall are used to expand the chest fully while breathing in and deflate it fully while breathing out. The chest and diaphragm are lifted up during inhalation and relaxed back down during exhalation. Most people breathe shallowly and quickly during normal life, using only their upper chest.

Shavasana A basic yoga pose, or asana, in which the body is totally relaxed and the mind still. It is performed lying flat on the back with the legs together but not touching, feet turned out, and arms lying flat close to the body with the palms up. The eyes should be closed, facial muscles relaxed, and breathing deep and slow.

Stress incontinence This is an involuntary loss of urine that occurs when there is raised pressure in the abdomen, perhaps from sneezing, coughing, laughing, or exercise. It can be due to weakened pelvic floor muscles or a weakened urethral sphincter.

Tadasana A standard yoga pose, or asana, often called the "mountain pose". The foundation standing pose, it is performed with the feet apart, weight pressing into the floor, and the arms hanging beside the body. The body should be relaxed and balanced, and the ankles, knees, hips, shoulders, and ears should be aligned.

Trikonasana A standard yoga pose, or asana, often called the "triangle pose". One of the fundamental standing poses of yoga, it is performed with legs straight and apart in the form of a triangle, with one foot turned outward and the upper body leaning down toward that side. The palm of the hand on that side rests flat on the floor for support. The other arm is raised to the ceiling and the head looks up.

Upanishads A series of ancient Hindu scriptures. The word "upanishad" means "to sit down near" and also "sacred and secret knowledge".

Whooshing An effective way to soothe a fretful baby. Hold your baby facing away from you with your arms resting under his seat and around his chest for support. Swing him from side to side in a rhythmic movement to suit his mood.

List of useful organizations

Association for Post-Natal Illness (APNI)
145 Dawes Road, Fulham,
London, SW6 7EB
Tel: 0207 386 0868
www.apni.org
Provides a national network of support for mothers suffering from postnatal illness.

Birthlight
PO Box 148, Cambridge, CB4 2GB
Tel: 01223 362288
www.birthlight.com
Provides a network of trained teachers in antenatal, postnatal, and baby yoga.

Bliss (The National Charity for the Newborn)
68 South Lambeth Road,
London, SW8 1RL
Tel: 0207 820 9567
www.bliss.org.uk
Offers advice, support, and information in connection with newborn babies needing special health care.

British Wheel of Yoga
1 Hamilton Place, Boston Road,
Seaford, Lincs, NG34 7ES
Tel: 01592 303233
www.bwy.org.uk
A member organization of yoga teachers in the UK.

Contact A Family
209–211 City Road,
London, EC1V 1JN
Tel: 0207 7608 8700
www.cafamily.org.uk
Offers support and advice to families with disabled children or children with specific health conditions.

Gingerbread
7 Sovereign Court, Sovereign Close,
London, E1W 2HW
Tel: 0207 488 9300
www.gingerbread.org.uk
Offers information, advice, and support to lone parents through a network of local groups.

Home-Start
2 Salisbury Road, Leicester, LE1 7QR
Tel: 0116 233 9955
www.home-start.org.uk
Volunteers offer support and practical help to families with at least one child under five years old.

International Association of Infant Massage
PO Box 247, Rainham,
Essex, RM13 7WT
Tel: 01279 319896
www.iam.org.uk
Provides information on local infant massage classes.

La Leche League (Great Britain)
PO Box 29, West Bridgford,
Nottingham, NG2 7NP
Tel: 0845 120 2918
www.laleche.org.uk
Supports mothers with breastfeeding challenges.

Meet a Mum Association (MAMA)
Tel: (helpline) 0208 768 0123
www.leguer.demon.co.uk
Provides support, information, and help to women suffering from postnatal depression.

National Childbirth Trust (NCT)
Alexandra House, Oldham Terrace,
Acton, London, W3 6NH
Tel: 0870 770 3236
www.nctpregnancyandbabycare.com
Provides local postnatal support and information.

Parentline Plus
Tel: (helpline) 0800 800 2222
www.parentlineplus.org.uk
Offers support to anyone parenting a child.

Serene (Incorporating the Cry-Sis helpline)
BM Cry-Sis, 27 Old Gloucester Street,
London, WC1N 3XX
Tel: 0207 404 5011
Provides support to families with excessively crying, sleepless, or demanding babies and young children.

SureStart
Level 2, Caxton House, Tothill Street,
London, SW1H 9NA
Tel: 0870 0002288
www.surestart.gov.uk
Aims to provide for the physical, intellectual, and social development of pre-school children.

The Yoga Theraph Centre
90–92 Pentonville Road,
London, N1 9HS
Tel: 0207 689 3040
www.yogatherapy.org
The Yoga Biomedical Trust for yoga therapy, pregnancy yoga and mother and baby yoga.

Recommended reading

General yoga

Asana Pranayama Mudra Bandha
Swami Satyananda Saraswati. Yoga Publications Trust, Munger, Bilhar, India, 2002

Breath – The Essence of Yoga, A Guide to Inner Stillness
Sandra Sabatini. Thorsons, London, 2000

The Complete Illustrated Guide to Ayurveda – The Ancient Indian Healing Tradition
Gopi Warrier and Deepika Gunawant. Element Books Limited, Shaftsbury, Dorset, 1997

Yoga, Mind, Body and Spirit, A Return to Wholeness
Donna Farhi. Henny Holt and Company, New York, 2000

Specialist yoga

Beat Fatigue With Yoga.
The Simple Step by Step Way to Restore Energy
Fiona Agombar. Thorsons, London, 2002

Fly Like a Butterfly (Yoga for Children)
Shakta Kaur Khalsa. Rudra Press, Canada, 1998

Yoga for Wellness.
Healing With the Timeless Teachings of Vini Yoga
Gary Kraftsow. Penguin Arkana, Arkana, 1999

Yoga – A Gem for Women
Geeta Iyengar. Allied Publishers Limited, New Delhi, 2000

Mother and Baby Yoga

Baby Yoga
Françoise Barbira Freedman. Gaia Books Limited, London, 2000

Post-natal Yoga
Françoise Barbira Freedman. Lorenz Books, London, 2000

Baby massage

Infant Massage, A Handbook for Loving Parents
Vimala McClure. Souvenir Press, New York, 2003

Loving Hands – The Traditional Art of Baby Massage
Frederic Leboyer. Collins, London, 1977

Child development and parenting

Emotional Intelligence. Why It Can Matter More than IQ
Daniel Goleman. Bloomsbury Publishing, London, 1996

Emotionally Intelligent Parenting. How to Raise a Self-Disciplined, Responsible, Socially Skilled Child
Maurice Elias, Steven Tobias, and Brian Friedlander. Hodder and Stoughton, London, 1988

Natural Childbirth –
A Practical Guide to the First Seven Years
John B. Thomson. Gaia Books Limited, London, 1994

The Sleep Book for Tired Parents!
Help Solving Childrens' Sleep Problems
Rebecca Huntley. Parenting Press, Seattle, 1991; Souvenir Press, London, 1992

Birthing Traditions

Rediscovering Birth
Sheila Kitzinger. Little Brown and Company (UK), London, 2000

Index

Author's acknowledgements

I would like to thank the team at Mitchell Beazley for their help – especially to Vivienne, John, Sally, Tim, Nicky, Victoria, and Deirdre. Thank you Ruth for your patience and smiles, Vicky for modelling and teaching me about make-up! A huge thank you to all my models – mothers and babies who appeared in the book and to my St Albans mums who helped me out with the presentations.

Thank you to my teachers: Andrea Wilson; Francoise Freedman of "Birthlight"; Robin Munro from the Yoga Therapy Centre, and Ralph who has taught me the true meaning of yoga.

Thank you St Albans "Costa-Cafe" who allowed me to write for hours in their cafe without buying a coffee. Thank you Giles who cared for the children while I wrote.

But most of all, thank you to my kids; it's not easy living with a mother!

Commissioning Editor Vivienne Antwi
Art Director Tim Foster
Designer Victoria Burley
Production Faizah Malik
Photographer Ruth Jenkinson
Copy Editor Anne McDowall
Proofreader Alyson Lacewing
Index Ann Parry